From **Lad**
to **Dad**

From Lad to Dad

The ultimate guide to pregnancy for blokes

Stephen Giles

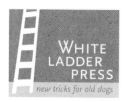

WHITE
LADDER
PRESS
new tricks for old dogs

From Lad to Dad

This edition first published in Great Britain 2008 by
Crimson Publishing, a division of Crimson Business Ltd
Westminster House
Kew Road
Richmond
Surrey
TW9 2ND

A catalogue record for this book is available from the British library.

ISBN 978 1 905410 40 8

Designed and typeset by Julie Martin Ltd
Cover design by Julie Martin Ltd
Cover photography by Judy Hedger
Printed and bound by Mega Printing, Turkey

To my Dad

Acknowledgements

This book wouldn't have been possible without the help and support of a number of people – above all Elle and 'the boy'. I'd also like to thank David Burke and Steve Fountain for their time and criticism, and the surveyed fathers for their help in providing new and surprising angles. Finally, thanks to Roni and Rich at White Ladder for making the idea work.

Contents

Introduction
Welcome to Planet Dad

Welcome to a new world. It's a place where the breasts are bigger, the bank balances are smaller and where you're surrounded by people talking in a language you don't understand. Much like being on a package holiday really.

And as a smart traveller, what you need is a first-rate guide book to get you through – to show you the shortcuts and the pitfalls. You need simple and clear explanations of the new landscape and just enough of the lin go to get you around. You need the essentials – information on sex, relationships, money, health and what to do in an emergency. And this is what you'll find in these pages, written by someone who has been there, done it, bought the T-shirt and then had a baby vomit all over it.

This book will give the support you need to travel through the next nine months without stepping on anyone's toes along the way – from the doubts and fears you might have before your baby is even conceived, through the strange and sometimes freakish world of pregnancy and medical care to the unknown horrors of the delivery suite and that unbelievable moment when you finally get your hands on the new life you helped to create.

This is not just another guide to supporting your partner; it sets out to help specifically with your emotional and practical needs. Sure, some of those are going to help her too, but she's got a lot of people on her team – you're the one who could be left with the feeling that you're completely and utterly alone.

In fact, that might be just what you're going through right now, depending on how far you are along the road. Alone, thrilled, scared, jealous, overwhelmed, intimidated, excited, anxious – we've all been there and if we haven't been there yet, we'll get there soon.

But often these important emotions get ignored as the dad-to-be is sidelined and stereotyped by medical staff or by relatives and friends who stick to another old-fashioned belief – that pregnancy is all about the woman. Is that fair? Well, it's true that she's got the physical burden, but frankly you've still got to live with her, to cope with the physical and emotional changes that she's going through. Most of all, you've got to turn yourself into a father, to learn how to be responsible for another life that depends on you for its existence – and that's not going to happen overnight.

So this is both a personal and practical story of pregnancy from a man's viewpoint. The personal part comes in the shape of the journal which I kept immediately before and during my wife's pregnancy with our first child. It draws on my experiences and those of people I spoke to at the time. It is totally honest, which is a cop out way of excusing all the stupid comments, outbursts and moments of sheer desperation that I reckon I must have shared with most men in my position.

The practical aspect of the book is in two parts. First, it's in the advice that helped me through this momentous time. While putting together material for this book I discovered a tonne of shared experience and frustration among fathers-to-be. I have added as much as I can, not with cast-iron answers but with suggestions of things that worked for me, and for others.

The second practical part of this book comes in the form of snippets of information that I found useful, or that I would have loved to have known at the time. These also draw heavily on the feedback gained from a survey of new and expectant fathers which was carried out for this book – and which gave me access to a wide cross section of knowledge and advice. Some of the best quotes and thoughts from new dads are included along the way. My thanks go out to everyone who helped make this a truly broad sweep of experience.

Of course, everyone's experience of pregnancy is unique. But because of the way fathers-to-be tend to get viewed in our society, you may be coming to this book feeling a bit isolated, maybe even a bit lost and detached from the whole pregnancy. I guarantee you won't leave it with that feeling. Here is the proof that you are not alone. Nor are you useless, powerless or redundant. You're the daddy, almost. And absolutely nothing beats that.

Chapter One
Trying for a baby

"I realised early on that life with a baby will forever be a 'we' life, not an 'I' life." R, dad of one.

I blame Christmas. It's meant to be a harmless holiday, but it's actually a cover for dark forces who want to keep the planet filled with babies. Happy, childless couples all over the world get together with their families to have the same sentences banged into them – 'Christmas is for the kids' and 'children help to make sense of it all'.

Yeah, yeah, I get the picture. The oldies are tired of trying to make the day magical for their cynical grown-up kids. It's not much fun trying to photograph the look of inno-cent delight on the face of your goatee-bearded, marketing manager son as he unwraps his novelty latte set. I see why the ancients want a grandchild to take up the wide-eyed role in this nonsense.

But do they have to be so ball-crushingly obvious about it? Nothing puts you off shagging so much as your parents expecting it of you. This year, for some reason, they have forgotten their duty to remind us to get down to it for the sake of future Christmases. Which, naturally, made us think seriously about starting a family.

Elle and I have been together for about eight years, married for six, and pretty happy. The idea of a family has always been at the fringe of our relationship. We've followed the familiar route of buying cats and then treating them like children – albeit children who shit in a box. We even bought dogs and treated them like children – albeit children who shag pillows and eat cat shit. But, until now, coping with the disgusting habits of our pets has been enough of a distraction to keep the idea of real children at bay.

Now we'll be put off no longer. We're committed to it, one hundred per cent. But it's just words at this stage, which means it's pretty easy to be blasé about the whole deal.

• • •

Maybe not. Just a few days have passed since we agreed to start trying and already the pressure is creeping into our sex life. I've been coming up with pro and con lists in my head. I'm not really worried about the baby, because that's so far away I can't take it in. I'm more concerned that, whatever happens as a result of our 'trying', my life is going to change.

Scenario one is that Elle doesn't become pregnant for ages. I've heard it can take around two years to do the business. What if it takes us longer? I'm not old, not really old, but I will be in, say, five years. I've already started to take an unhealthy interest in those magazine ads for book clubs and I've started hanging around near the slippers in shoe shops.

Worse than that is the fear of what failing to conceive could do for our sex life. I'm pleased to say that I've always found sex to be fun, spontaneous and, well, sexy. Bringing in thermometers, leg clamps and astral charts would surely be very, very bad news. I don't want to have to start worrying about what pants to wear or how hot my bath water should be. Then there's those horrible checks of bodily functions. If they find out I've got a low sperm count will I regret wasting so much of it as a teenager?

We've got friends who've been trying for a baby for a while and the wait does seem to have a big effect on them, emotionally and physically. I admire their persistence, but their sex lives have got all of the glamour and excitement of a Star Trek convention. What if the long wait for a baby changes things, particularly our relationship? Will we start to resent each other if it doesn't happen? And what about the cost of doing things medically if we can't manage it naturally?

The Sperminator

How to boost your sperm count

If you want to increase the odds of conceiving there are a few tried and tested methods that can get the little fellows swimming en masse.

Stop smoking and cut down on the booze. All drugs lower your sperm count, so cut down on caffeine too.

Box clever. Wearing boxer shorts instead of tight-fitting pants keeps your testes cool and maximises the chances of sperm production.

Have a cold shower. Or at least a cool bath. Avoiding extremes of temperature is another sure-fire way to make the most of your sperm production.

It seems a bit bleak to worry about years of miserable waiting right at the start of what is meant to be a fantastic experience. But it's just like travelling on British trains, you need to forget about the destination, what counts is surviving the journey. If we aren't capable of handling frustration and failure then we aren't ready to try.

Till birth us do part?

Testing your relationship

When you're trying for a baby the spotlight may be on your performance in the bedroom, but it's also a time of serious pressure on your whole relationship. Whether you hit the jackpot first time or spend years trying, the result is hopefully the same – a baby. But to get through the journey you and your partner have got to be one hell of a strong unit, otherwise you'll fail. We've all heard plenty of stories about couples 'staying together for the children', or 'having a baby to save a relationship' and the one common link in all these cases is that it doesn't work. Which is why now is the time to ask yourself the serious, searching questions you need answering about your relationship, not after the event. When you have a baby it is a tie, something linking you and your partner together for life, so you've got to be extra sure that this commitment is right for you. Can you honestly picture yourself with her in 20 years? If you're having doubts, and you don't feel right chatting it through with your mates or your family, have a confidential chat with a relationship counselling service like Relate – you'll find them online and in the phone book – the peace of mind is worth the effort. The more secure you are that this is the right way forward, the more relaxed you will be later in the pregnancy, when the stress rises and your relationship can be seriously tested.

Scenario two is much more frightening. What if Elle gets pregnant before we're ready? OK, before I'm ready. And how the hell am I supposed to know that I am ready?

The biggest question in this scenario is what would change if she became pregnant? Would I suddenly be unable to jet off to South Africa to take part in the bridge jumping championships? Would my career as a professional water-skier fail before I've had the chance to pull on my first wetsuit? Would I age prematurely and would my politics swing wildly to the right? Probably.

In truth, my life isn't so dramatic that a baby would spoil things for me. The closest I ever get to dangerous sport is running with scissors. In fact, I'm a bit of a lazy bastard and no amount of trying to pass off my beer gut as puppy fat will make me seem younger. When it comes to being a dad I suppose I'm as ready as I'll ever be. But that doesn't mean I want to admit it to myself just yet.

Excess baggage

Freedom and the new arrival

Here's a tip for you – sit down and making a list of all the things you've done in the last five years – all the holidays you've taken, all the last minute getaways you've fitted in. Then put a tick against each one you wouldn't be able to manage with a baby. Repeat the exercise for things you've always wanted to do but haven't managed.

I guarantee that, at least when it comes to travelling, you're a lot more flexible with a nipper in tow than you thought. A mate of mine has just returned from a cross Africa trek with his young family, and others have chalked up trips to Morocco, Jordan, South America and the wildest recesses of Canada. Sure, it takes a bit more planning, and the bags are a bit heavier, but you don't need to start booking through special-ist, expensive agents, or putting yourself through the hell of Disney every year – just go direct to the hotels and resorts you plan to visit – most are now online and incredibly easy to deal with. It's the best way to be sure you're getting what you want. It is usually an awful lot cheaper, too.

. . .

A couple of weeks into the new year and already life is different. I've never considered myself to be a particularly attractive man. I'm not ugly, but I don't have the smooth beauty of a movie star or the rough charm of a rugby player. I look more like a movie star who's just played a particularly nasty rugby match. Yet my wife has never found me more sexually attractive. If trying for a baby is going to turn into a shag-fest, maybe it would be better if we let it run for a couple of years.

Elle's hormones are leaping around all over the place at the moment, but I haven't experienced much change. Except for the whole sex slave thing, of course. We got even more practice in during our weekend away to celebrate our anniversary, though my efforts to produce a baby were probably ended by the huge amount of alcohol I drank.

Drinking a lot is a near unconscious way of saying that I'm not coping too well with the idea of becoming a dad. To be honest I'm shitting myself at the possibility. The drink doesn't help there, either. Any way up it's a bad move, and they also say that too much alcohol has a negative effect on fertility. Is this my mind at work, trying to stop us getting anywhere?

I think about the baby a lot now. Whenever we go out for a drink, or the cinema, or just out to the shops, I try to picture a little bundle of screams and tears with its pile of nappy bags and huge off-roader push chair, and I wonder whether we'd ever be able to do the things that we enjoy again. I can cope with losing the big things in life – like that two-seater sports cars I always wanted – but I don't know that I can cope without the simple things like the odd pint and a wander round town.

Reality hit hard on the way home from our anniversary weekend when Elle said she 'felt pregnant'. She didn't offer this as a matter of fact, we haven't been trying long enough to know whether she's even missed a period yet. It's just instinct, another example of her shift to some higher mental plane, while I'm still just relishing the extra sex. She was keen to test her theory.

Feeling a bit self-conscious, we stopped at a supermarket some miles from home to buy a pregnancy test kit. This brought memories flooding back of buying my first packet of condoms. It still feels naughty to admit that, though we've been together some years, we are actually having sex. At least I didn't park in the 'parent and child' spaces.

Testing, testing, 1, 2, 3

How to handle pregnancy tests

Tricky one, the pregnancy test. The tests themselves come in a range of shapes and sizes, most commonly a little white stick that looks like an electric toothbrush which your partner pisses over. It's better if she doesn't do this in the dark, in a room with other electric toothbrushes. The tricky bit is whether this is something you should get involved with at all. Our surveyed dads were split on the issue – though the words of one sums it all up neatly, 'trust your partner's instincts'.

If she wants to involve you with the test, that's great, but you need to be able to cope with the despair of a negative result. If she wants to do the thing in her own time, maybe she thinks it would be easier to cope with a negative result without sharing it with you. That may or may not be true, so keep an eye out just in case she needs a bit of support after a negative test. And always check your electric toothbrush carefully.

Whatever she wants to do, don't take offence and don't push it. There's no right or wrong way to handle tests, just the way that suits her. You've got to be ready with the bubbly or with tissues, to be able to celebrate, console or just keep silent. Told you it was tricky.

As soon as we got home Elle disappeared into the bathroom and I paced the floor like a 1950s caricature, longing for a pipe stem to chew. As I paced, I looked around me and tried to imagine our tiny home being invaded by a noisy, demanding child.

Our little house is pretty basic, just about big enough for the pair of us. I could hear the neighbours crashing pots and pans in their kitchen the other side of the thin wall. I pictured their angry thumps on the same thin wall as the baby launched into another 3am screaming fit.

This is too bleak, I decided, as the toilet flushed and broke my train of thought. Try to focus on the wonderful reality of fatherhood, the joy of creating a unique life, full of potential. Think positive.

"Well?" I said, trying not to show my own conflict.

"Negative," she sighed.

"Never mind," I said, holding her. Inside I was relieved, not because I hadn't wanted her to be happy, but because I hadn't expected my response to the test to be so uncertain. I can't believe that I've come so near to creating a new life while still questioning the whole idea of trying for a baby in the first place.

A life sentence?

Making sense of the future

Making a new life is the closest any of us will come to playing God, so it's no surprise some of us get a bit stressed out by the idea. It opens up a whole set of deep questions – should I bring a child into the world, is it just selfishness? Do I want one because Kevin from Accounts has got one? Does the planet really need another mouth to feed? Of course it does. OK, so Mr and Mrs Hitler should have just watched a video instead, but for every rotten egg there's a Gandhi or even a Wayne Rooney (though hopefully better looking).

It's like pulling a cracker – you don't know what you're going to get, but without the bang you'll never find out. Of course, not every dad-to-be gets the chance to think too deeply about such big issues, a fair few pregnancies are surprises, to both mum and dad. It can be a bit hard to take that you've created this incredible thing without any serious planning. In fact, nothing can make you feel more cut off from the pregnancy.

But it is still important to go through these thoughts and fears, even if the baby is already on its way. Shutting them out because the result is inevitable won't work, and there aren't many worries that can't be dealt with between you and your partner. Playing God means being responsible, but at this stage that just means being true to yourself, so look at what worries you and make sure you deal with it.

• • •

The negative test has made Elle a bit more thoughtful too. In the weeks since she took the test, we haven't talked about it as much as we should, mainly because I'm frightened of creating an 'issue'. The more we discuss it, the more it will become a matter of stress and that's going to be bad. But she's an impatient person and she's also used to being in control. The idea that her body can play tricks on her has come as a bit of a shock.

It may be this shock to the system that's making her ill. She's been totally run down for a while and we're off on holiday in a few days to the Highlands of Scotland. I'm hoping that the heady combination of winter sun, sea, sand, sex and scotch will help her. At least it'll give us the chance to talk about things, and it might give me the opportunity to get my head around the idea of babies.

Just a couple of months in and I can already see how important it is to limit stress while trying for a baby. Anything that threatens the future becomes a real problem, which is bad news as Elle works in a pretty depressed manufacturing sector and my income as a freelance writer is patchy at best. So we're not exactly big on financial stability. If we let work worries crowd our lives then it'll be even harder to allow time for baby making, but if we don't worry enough about work we won't provide a secure platform for the future.

So how much stress is OK and how much will harm our attempts at conception? All the medical advice suggests that too much stress reduces our chance of doing the business. It seems like such a delicate balancing act – no wonder they call it the miracle of birth.

. . .

Until today our Scottish holiday has been relaxing and quiet. Our evenings have been marked by huge meals which I have attacked with all the enthusiasm of a fat bastard while Elle has pushed the deep-fried haggis around her plate as if it was, well, deep-fried haggis.

She's maintained that she's alright, and she hasn't seemed too bad, except for the lack of appetite, but I know her well enough to be sure something's wrong. This morning, as we drove the hundred miles or so to our final hotel of the tour, we finally talked about it.

Rather than having a lot of worries that were making her ill, Elle's biggest fear was the illness itself. Running through the symptoms, she started worrying about the reasons for her loss of appetite, her tiredness and lack of energy.

We'd got as far as that beautiful bit of landscape that's been spoiled forever by some arsehole of a council official sticking up 'Monarch of the Glen country' signs everywhere when Elle, who had been lost in her thoughts for a few minutes, turned to me.

"I could have something really horrible," she said.

"No," I assured her.

"There is another possibility," she added. "I could be pregnant."

I immediately though about the failed test, but, in a rare moment of tact, I held myself back from pointing this out. However small the hope of pregnancy might have been, it was possible, and any hope was better than her alternative.

So we stopped at a chemists, bought another kit – without giggling like school kids this time – and headed for the hotel. We dumped our bags and Elle headed straight for the bathroom. I began to pace up and down once more and tried to work out what I was going to say to console her when the inevitable disappointment came.

A couple of minutes later she came out of the bathroom with a strange smile. She didn't say a word, just stood back and let me through the door. The tiny testing kit, like a junior chemistry set, was spread over the tiled surface. Elle held up the test and the instructions. I looked at the pictures and back at the little strip. Positive. Pregnant. And about to change everything, forever.

In the circumstances, there was only one thing I could say. Bending closer to the tiny beaker of amber liquid, I nodded. "I've not seen your pee before."

What's happening?
The whole nine months

Life is about to change. The hard work starts now, not just in terms of the emotional and physical changes your partner is going to experience, but in the difference it will make to your own life and to your relationship.

This is the time to take stock of what you face in terms of changes and challenges ahead. Each chapter of this book will talk you through a month in the life of the pregnancy, explaining what will happen to your partner and your baby. But for those of you who need to know what happens as soon as you start reading a book, here's a very short summary of the whole process, broken down by month:

Month one.

Your partner's symptoms – very few noticeable symptoms or changes in mood or behaviour. Some women claim to have an 'instinct' that they are pregnant, but there are no real outward signs until after the first month. The first sign is a missed period.

Your baby – at less than 2mm long, your baby resembles a miniature shrimp. Don't worry, there's a long way to go.

Your role – relax, you don't even know about it yet.

Month two.

Your partner's symptoms – ranges from woman to woman, but as her body is slowly taken over by pregnancy hormones she may well be feeling sick or pre-menstrual, she may have tender or sore breasts, food cravings, mood swings, skin problems and constipation.

Your baby – by the end of month two, your baby is around 25mm and is actually beginning to resemble a tiny human.

Your role – provider of reassurance and comfort, strength and support. You'll need to hold her hair while she's sick, hold her hand while she's crying uncontrollably for no reason and hold everything else together while she readjusts to life with a baby inside her.

Month three.

Your partner's symptoms – she may start to gain a little weight and her abdomen will begin to alter to prepare for carrying the baby. Morning sickness may ease and her skin may clear up.

Your baby – by the end of this month genitals are forming and the baby is breathing and swallowing. The main organs are fully formed.

Your role – depends on the seriousness of her symptoms, but is likely still to involve a great degree of fetching, carrying, cooking and cleaning as she will still be incredibly tired a lot of the time.

Month four.

Your partner's symptoms – nipples become darker, abdomen grows, heart increases in size and efficiency. Skin begins to soften and 'bloom'.

Your baby – standing at a strapping 160mm, your baby is now capable of hearing, so be careful about swearing near your partner. Legs are fully formed.

Your role – it's possible you can relax a little around now. Your partner's energy will return and this will give you the breathing space to start thinking about things like work/life balance and how you're going to afford the whole thing in the first place.

Month five.

Your partner's symptoms – a complete loss of waistline, more awkwardness in movement and possibly even difficulty in sleeping all point to the fact that the baby is growing fast and your partner's body is having to adapt quickly to keep up.

Your baby – the little trooper is now 250mm and may be moving sufficiently for kicks and jabs to be felt by your partner.

Your role – supporter in a range of medical situations, at tests for abnormalities (from 15 weeks onwards) and anatomy scans (from around 20 weeks). You could try to make your increasingly uncomfortable partner more relaxed with massage.

Month six.

Your partner's symptoms – the baby's kicks will feel stronger and more frequent, your partner may also feel slight 'tightening' sensations known as Braxton Hicks contractions, don't worry, it's not the real thing. The sheer size of her uterus may be causing digestive issues like heartburn, stitches and breathlessness.

Your baby – heart is beating strongly and clearly, hearing is developing and the baby will respond to music and other audio stimuli.

Your role – chief planner at this stage. While your partner is still mobile, you might need to take the lead in a few shopping trips to select some of the baby essentials.

Month seven.

Your partner's symptoms – stretch marks may be visible around the abdomen as your partner's weight increases at pace. This will have a knock-on effect on her sleep and will also cause her to need the toilet more.

Your baby – the skin is becoming opaque and the eyes are starting to open and function.

Your role – you need to get back into the role of slave as your partner finds everyday tasks that much harder again. It's also a good time to organise any necessary DIY jobs that need doing.

Month eight.

Your partner's symptoms – she's now in countdown mode, and her brain may be elsewhere. It's possible that the baby's head may engage in the pelvis during this period, which will make breathing much easier for your partner.

Your baby – now almost fully formed and measuring a gargantuan 450mm, your baby is now extremely likely to cope with life outside the womb. But let's hope it stays there a while longer.

Your role – attend ante-natal classes to help yourself prepare for your part in the delivery room, make sure all the attendant worries – visitors in the hospital, parking, overnight bags etc – are dealt with so that your partner can relax for the final few weeks.

Month nine.

Your partner's symptoms – there's a wide range of possibilities, depending on how 'easy' the pregnancy has been. If you partner has had a rough time, she'll probably be feeling tired, irritable and utterly fed up with the whole experience. If it's been fairly straightforward, she may have a burst of energy pre-birth which carries her into the delivery suite. When she gets there she may well be on a different plane to you – partly because of pain and partly because of drugs.

Your baby – is full birth-weight and about to make an appearance.

Your role – bag carrier, supporter, sponge for all the abuse and insults you can take, chief photographer, breaker of the good news to relatives, security guard and, oh yes, dad.

Chapter Two
She's pregnant

"The day I first discovered I was going to be a dad was a fantastic, life-changing moment." G, dad of two

What's happening?

Month two.

Your partner's symptoms – this is the month when pregnancy really takes hold of your partner, introducing a whole range of symptoms that might take her, and you, by surprise. Hormonal changes are beginning to kick in and these affect appetite, digestion, balance, mood and energy levels, so don't be surprised if she feels a bit like she's been hit by a steam roller. One thing to look out for at the beginning of month two is what is known as an 'implantation' bleed, when the embryo attaches itself to the wall of the uterus and some old blood is disturbed. This can sometimes produce a small 'bleed' or spots of blood from your partner's vagina. Don't over-react to this, it's perfectly natural. For more information on bleeding in pregnancy see chapter four.

Your baby – at first glance your month-old embryo is a bit of a blob, but closer inspection reveals incredible detail even at this stage. Eyes, ears and essential organs are all in place, and while they're not all functioning yet, everything is coming together. The heart is working and the intestines are already processing nourishment. Ok, so its still a long way from getting out in the world and earning a decent living, but for an inch-high being, that's pretty impressive stuff.

I am a god. I'm Hercules. I'm Cristiano Ronaldo's right foot. I am Superman. I'm a caveman. I am the Walrus. Without wishing to underestimate Elle's involvement, I did it. Me. I decided to have a child and I've sodding well done it. First time, no questions asked, back of the net. Fantastic, fan-bloody-tastic. I am a sex machine. Out of my way, you puny mortals, for I am The Procreator.

I'm feeling a little drunk.

• • •

I feel better now. God it's been a strange day, from fear to disbelief to ecstasy and then all the way back to fear again.

For most of the day I've been basking in the sheer delight of knowing that I can do it. This feeling has nothing to do with the realities of impending parenthood, but I don't give a shit. I've just enjoyed being singularly, unashamedly masculine. It's a feeling of complete power, of wanting to hunt and gather, or at the very least order something off the room service menu.

It's an odd feeling, and as the unreal edge has worn off, I've started to feel a bit queasy. Back in the days of terraced football grounds, you could be swept up by a wave of fans charging forwards to celebrate a goal, or sideways to start a scrap. There was nothing you could do about it, and if you were pushed into a metal hurdle or a concrete pillar then that was your hard luck for standing too close. All afternoon, I've been surfing helplessly on the tide of events, but now I'm on the lookout for the concrete post of reality.

"Darling, I'm... petrified"

Reacting to the news

This might sound weird, but fairly common feelings dads-to-be go through just after getting the good news include shock, bewilderment and despair. Nothing actually prepares you for the moment, even if you've had years to get ready. Part of this strange feeling might come from the fact that it marks the end of your practical input, and the beginning of a new and bollock-shrinkingly scary part of a journey which you no longer control. You're expected to be excited and delighted, yet at the back of your mind are all the things that could go wrong that you can't do a sodding things to stop.

For me, it was literally a life changing moment, more than my 'I do' or even my signature on the mortgage agreement. And that's a hell of a lot to take in at once. So don't worry about a few negative feelings at this stage, just as long as they are balanced by the positives they are a big part of getting yourself ready for the rockier parts of what's to come.

My mood has hardened like concrete this evening. Until now we've ordered a bottle of wine with dinner each evening of the holiday and Elle has sipped a half glass without much enjoyment while I've downed the rest. Now we know the cause of her 'illness' I can't help feeling an expectation that the wine should go from the table altogether, a sign of my support and commitment to the pregnancy.

It should. But, though I'm keen to show my support, I also want to show that I'm going to stay the same. Life is about to change all around me, roles, responsibilities and plans are all set to be thrown up into the air and I need something to keep me steady in this new world order. Necking cheap wine is a pretty crappy way to stay steady, but it works for me – or at least it did tonight. In the end, I ordered it, Elle refused it, I drank it, along with a couple of whiskies and a beer or two for good measure. Now I feel shit, sick and excited at the same time.

Cigarettes and alcohol

Changing your habits

This is another bugger of a decision – one which split our surveyed dads into two camps. On one side are men who rush into pregnancy as if they're on some kind of health crusade, out go all the fags and booze and for some they don't even reappear after the birth. Most prefer to limit the fags if not the alcohol, and some brave souls decide that's it's a matter of independence so they don't give up a single smoke or a drop of hard stuff.

The only way to decide for yourself is to take a good look at the facts and then go for whatever your conscience tells you.

What we know for sure is that if you smoke near your partner, it might affect the health of the baby, and while drinking may not be any good for you, at least it doesn't have any direct effect on the nipper. So if you want a drink, drink. If you want to smoke, accept the health risk or go outside.

It's harder for your partner. She can't step away from the baby for a fag break, but she might cause real harm by carrying on. At the same time, she might get seriously stressed if she has to give up. And if she is giving up and you aren't, you're probably going to be doubling the stress on her.

The official line is that giving up smoking is the best gift a mother can give her baby, and that's not a bad way of looking at it from your perspective too. If you want to kick the weed, but need some moral support, check out Stop Smoking, Stay Cool (White Ladder) for a totally realistic and non-patronising account of kicking the habit.

Drinking is the same story, really. Again, try and be sensitive – if you're nailing pint after pint and she's sipping her fifth lemonade of the evening, you're going to get the bollocking you richly deserve. Easing off the sauce shows you care and that you're supporting her in what is a pretty miserable time, but it also has the serious advantage of working out one hell of a lot cheaper than being on the lash all the time.

Whether you save the money for a almighty bender once junior's born or just put it towards something for the nursery, you know your sacrifice isn't going waste. Which all adds up to Brownie points for you.

• • •

I woke up this morning sharing my bed with the mother of my child and the mother of all hangovers. To say I've been hit by the reality of the pregnancy is an understatement. I feel as if reality has dragged me from the comfort of my hotel, around to the back alley, where it has kicked the living shit out of me. As if that wasn't enough, it then forced me to drive to the grey, cold and unwelcoming city of Perth to look at baby clothes.

Baby shopping – what a nightmare. Two things are obvious straight away. Firstly, no matter how rich and successful I get, we'll never be able to afford to dress the poor little sod in anything more expensive than a brown paper bag. Secondly, we are the only people of child-bearing age who actually shop for clothes.

Mothers-in-law and elderly aunts hunt like packs of wolves for bootees and bibs, even reluctant grandpas linger with embarrassment around the romper suits, but no one of our age is anywhere to be seen. Where are these people and why aren't they buying clothes for their children? And why are they handing over this important task to freakish old people, capable of cooing over miniature tank tops?

One of these questions was answered at lunch. Because I'd been a good boy in the shops I was allowed fried chicken as compensation, so we headed for Perth's busiest fast food restaurant and squeezed into the luxury plastic seating next to a large family having some kind of kids' party.

It was hell. The adults were moody and irritable and their hideous children fought and squabbled like sewer rats while picking over the bones of the meal. Two toddlers squirmed in their buggies like convicts in the electric chair. One of these monsters was permanently whining –

a low, menacing, desolate soundtrack of misery to accompany our food. For the first time on record I didn't finish my chicken.

As we sat in the car I shook my head in disbelief at this nightmarish vision of the future. Elle looked across at me and smiled.

"They don't all end up like that," she said, but I couldn't work out if she was trying to convince me, or to convince herself.

"God, I hope not," I said. "I really hope not."

It really spooked me. I've spent this first day after the positive test wandering about in a complete daze, looking in horror and awe at dads with their kids and wondering what the hell I'm going to make of the whole business. I know there's nothing strange about this – it's part of the process of going from the theory of having a baby to the reality of becoming a father. But am I going to be as witless as some of the arseholes I've seen today? Will I be able to stop myself from forcing my views on the poor kid? Will I make them support my team and follow in my footsteps or will I force the little soul to become a lawyer or a doctor, or something else 'worthwhile'? Will I be a pushy dad or a laid-back dad? Will I be just like my own dad or the complete opposite?

Back at the hotel my fears for the future were put to one side. I decided that we needed to contact the doctor at home to get an appointment as soon as possible on our return. I am fairly sure that we've got to have some kind of medical tests before anything can be properly recognised, so we got the number and I got Elle to make the call.

Body talk

Changes and your partner

Your partner's body will be going through a huge cycle of emotional and physical changes about now – and these will continue for the whole of pregnancy and beyond. Men view the changes to their partner's body and mood with, at best, curiosity and at worst, revulsion. Most are at the very least surprised by the changes they see unfolding and expanding around them day-by-day, so you'd be well advised to have at least a working knowledge of her likely symptoms from day one. Forewarned is forearmed, they say. So here goes with a down-and-dirty survival guide for some of the most common changes and symptoms:

Morning sickness. This can, apparently, be a sickness that affects a woman in the morning. But it can also be a slight nausea that lasts all day, or a full-on vomit fest that only happens in aisle 5 of the super-market. It's normally a symptom of early pregnancy only, and usually fades away by about 12 to 14 weeks. Some women get a condition called hyperemesis, which is really bad sickness that lasts through the whole pregnancy and might need hospital treatment if things get real-ly bad. But for most women, it's usually pretty mild, and might be trig-gered at mealtimes, or by specific smells or tastes. Generally, your partner's senses are stronger, so any powerful or distinctive smell may cause her to heave.

Some women don't get sick at all, but if yours is blowing chunks how do you help her deal with it? The women who wake up, throw up and get on with the day actually seem to get off fairly light, as most of them appear to feel fine thereafter. There's not much you can do for them, except hold the toilet seat.

Elle's was a fairly mild but constant illness between about four and 10 weeks. She felt alright most of the time. But when she felt bad, she avoided food, and that isn't really the best option – eating and drink-ing little and often is a good answer with these milder symptoms. Get your partner to keep a few biscuits handy – ginger ones in particular seem to work well for many women.

Vaginal discharge. OK, so it's not exactly a subject for the dinner table, but discharges from the vagina are quite common in pregnancy although they are normally odourless and harmless. If the discharge is thicker and smelly it might be a sign of a vaginal infection and this can have an impact on you if you spend any time down there (see sex, chapter five). More importantly, it can be a source of worry for your partner, who may feel concerned about doing any sustained activity like long walks etc for fear of discharges. On top of this there is the real, although slight, concern that the discharge could be amniotic fluid from the uterus and may be a signal that there' a problem. This is only likely if there's a big gush of liquid and in this event, you need to get to the hospital to have her checked out.

Cravings. There aren't many women who actually eat coal smeared with marmalade, but strange cravings are fairly common. There's nothing really wrong with developing an obsession with a particular food group as long as she can be persuaded to eat from others as well. The main issues with cravings stem from a desire to eat food that's off the menu for pregnant women – unpasteurised cheeses, patés, seafood and nuts, or the rare but quite disturbing craving known as Pica, a desire to eat non-food items like soap or dirt. This might be viewed as harmless, even amusing, but it might be a front for a more serious complaint, so get it checked out by the doc.

Fainting, dizziness and tiredness. Some unkind individuals suggest that women's brains take a nine-month holiday when they become pregnant, which is a completely unfair an unfounded accusation. It's more like three months. Part of the reason that so many men write off their partners as being completely dizzy during pregnancy is because they actually are dizzy, as well as exhausted and stressed. Pregnancy hormones make things hard for your partner in many ways, and changes to her blood vessels may cause sudden dizzy spells as well as fainting. She should avoid standing for long periods (which means getting the mother-in-law to do the ironing) and should take extra care when getting up, as standing too quickly can cause serious giddiness.

Constipation, piles and wind. Mmm, nice. Just when you thought you were the only one with disgusting digestive habits, along comes pregnancy and turns your partner into someone who wouldn't look out of place on a rugby tour. All of these issues are common in pregnancy, caused by a combination of hormonal changes and physical changes. All can be relieved, in part at least, by a decent, fibre-rich diet and plenty of water. Until then, I'd suggest opening a window.

Stretch marks and varicose veins. When you're carrying a sizeable additional weight inside your body it is going to leave its mark on the skin and on those load-bearing legs. While neither stretch marks nor varicose veins are attractive, there's not a lot that can be done to guard against them or to eliminate them once they appear. So if you want to make your life a misery, complain about them, otherwise accept them for what they are – a badge of honour.

Swollen limbs and weight gain. While swollen limbs – hands, feet, fingers etc –are an inevitable side-effect of pregnancy that can be eased with rest, the amount of weight your partner gains in pregnancy may depend on many factors, including diet, exercise and her metabolism. It is not, however, essential that she gains as much weight as possible, whatever your mother says about eating for two. Weight gain isn't regarded as a serious indicator of progress in pregnancy so stuffing cake into your partner's mouth to push up her weight is just plain cruel.

On the flipside, some men find the idea of their partner gaining weight unappealing. Get over it, I say. She'll quickly lose a good deal of the weight after the birth in any case and if you want to push her into getting back to that perfect pre-pregnancy figure, maybe you should try getting back to the weight and fitness level of your 18 year old self first. No? Thought not.

This is the first time I have taken over and Elle, normally a strong-willed woman, just let me. It is only a small thing, but it's pretty scary – especially as my gut instinct that the doctor is the next step is based on things I've heard on TV and on a belief that as doctors, like butchers, are known by their surnames, they must be important.

If we are going to be led by this kind of half-arsed crap for the whole nine months, we are in some serious trouble.

Chapter Three
Making changes

"Try to understand things from her position as soon as you can – if not to help her then just to get up to speed with what's going on." V, dad of two

What's happening?

Month three

Your partner's symptoms – particular smells and tastes are still likely to give your partner problems as her body continues to respond to the hormonal changes going on inside. She may still be struggling with sickness and general lethargy. Don't worry, it will get better soon. On the plus side it should be becoming increasingly obvious that she is pregnant, not just because of the slight curve of her belly, but also because her breasts are swelling. This is all well and good, but it's also accompanied by tenderness, so go steady (see sex, chapter 5). The more her breasts grow in pregnancy, the more important it is that she gets decent support, so she will need to be fitted for a decent maternity bra in the latter half of pregnancy.

Your baby – the baby is now capable of moving around, although still so small that these movements can't be felt by the mother. With all the organs in place, your baby's prime priority now is to grow and thrive, everything from this stage onwards is just a case of getting bigger and stronger.

Now that the holiday's over, we've got to face up to the fact that our parents must be told. Elle thinks we should keep the baby a secret until it is around 16 years old. It's the only way to give the poor little sod a chance of getting away without having to wear knitted bonnets. That won't be easy, so the other choice is to tell the family early, which gives them a chance to calm down before the birth.

It should be a happy process, but we're really not looking forward to it. The first step is to stop off on the journey home and tell Elle's sister, who's been trying for a baby for a while, and who might be a bit pissed off by the news that we seem to have started a family almost without effort.

It is hard to step back from our excitement long enough to see that other people may have their own reasons for not celebrating with us. We could be selfish about it and argue that nothing counts beyond us and the baby, but that wouldn't get us very far.

"I've got some news"
Telling the world

Telling people your good news is another bit of emotional juggling. Our surveyed men were split again – half decided to tell family as soon as possible and half waited until 12 weeks to tell everyone. Only one of our blokes blabbed to everyone immediately, which shows that they're generally a patient lot, but also that there's quite a lot of other stuff to worry about in the first few weeks. You'll need to pull the same trick you managed with the pregnancy test – let your partner's instincts lead, but try and keep hold of the situation yourself.

If the worst happens and she loses the baby, everyone you've told will need to hear the bad news too. One in five pregnancies don't make it, but most of these end before 12 weeks, so holding back a bit now might save a load of pain later.

On a different and happier note, you should remember that 40 weeks of pregnancy is actually one hell of a long time. For most of that time you'll be getting your ear bent by a ton of unwanted advice and criticism from everyone ranging from close family to your next-door neighbours' cousin's boss. If you wait until 12 weeks to break the news you can enjoy the peace and quiet of secrecy for a little bit longer. It might give you the time to get your head around what you want to do before big Auntie Pat weighs in with what you should be doing.

Our visit to Elle's sister began pretty awkwardly. I stood in the living room, chatting about football with my brother-in-law while Elle went to help make lunch. After what seemed like ages, during which time I used up all my small talk and most of my big talk too, her sister called us through to the dining room. I tried to catch Elle's eye and she smiled but said nothing. I felt terrible. I had no idea whether Elle had told her, or whether there was about to be a huge scene.

"You're going to be an uncle," Elle's sister told her husband as he was sitting down, catching him off guard.

"Oh, right, congratulations," he said, probably wondering why the hell I hadn't mentioned that instead of banging on about Man United's shit defence. I wondered the same thing.

Back in the car, we were so relieved. The hard part had been done, and her sister had coped with the news brilliantly – whoever else we told, it would be a piece of piss. Yeah, right.

The next people to hear the news were Elle's parents, who'd been looking after the house and pets for us. We'd thought about this one, and planned a little ceremony in which we presented her dad with a flat cap – a symbol of his new grandpa status. We stood back and waited for their response.

Nothing happened. Her dad smiled the false smile of confused gratitude for a strange present, while he was probably wondering why we were being so rude after he'd given a week of his life to look after our pets.

A few moments later the penny dropped with Elle's mother. "You mean you're pregnant?" she cried, as we breathed big sighs of relief and nodded. Then the congratulations came flooding out and he smiled with genuine delight.

After all that nonsense, I decided to just ring my parents

and break the news – needless to say it was one hell of a lot easier.

• • •

All of Elle's holiday health problems checked out as normal for early pregnancy during today's visit to the doctor. I was crapping myself about this visit, I'd cleared the morning in case tests and examinations went on for a while. We even arrived early, so that we'd appear keen.

Why the hell did we bother? It was all over in five minutes. So what did I expect? Well, I thought there'd be some kind of confirmation – the doctor's supposed to be a nice old guy who leans across his big oak desk, shakes me by the hand, gives me a cigar and says 'congratulations, Mr Giles, you're going to be a father'.

Yet our GP couldn't have been more different. Firstly she was a woman and secondly she just took our positive test as evidence of the pregnancy. She didn't even say 'well done'. No handshake, nothing. She just asked a few questions, checked blood pressure, examined Elle and gave a short talk on what Elle should and shouldn't eat.

We were given a form to fill in which registers Elle for

antenatal care, and sent on our way. We stood at the reception desk feeling gutted and looking like a couple who've just had some really bad news.

Now the whole experience seems even less real than it was before. All we have is a positive pregnancy test – actually we've now done three positive pregnancy tests, just to be on the safe side – and the medical profession are offering nothing more than the promise of a trip to the midwife in a month or so. What the hell am I supposed to do while we wait? What if I do something horribly wrong? Should I force Elle to stay indoors, in bed, until it's all over?

Have we been short-changed? Even my parents – during the now daily phone calls – seemed upset that we didn't have more to tell them after this appointment, and they must have been through the same thing.

The phone seems to ring almost all the time these days. After a quick enquiry about my health, my mum/ her mum/ her sister asks to speak to Elle, desperate to listen to the tiniest detail about how she is. Only a few people know that Elle is pregnant, yet they've already managed to make me feel like a total outsider. And that's just the women – I haven't even spoken to my dad yet, but Elle's dad already has the air of someone who expects his son-in-law to get a proper job, shave regularly and start looking after his little girl and, more importantly, his first grand-child.

I'm feeling a bit jealous, to tell the truth. I don't see why this pregnancy is only about Elle. There was a lot of hard work on my part too. Well, a bit. The phrase 'we're pregnant' has always made me want to throw up, mainly because it sounds like a line from one of those American made-for-TV movies but also because it shows a total ignorance of biology. But I can understand it a little better now. For better or worse I am a part of this experience, though right now it feels as if I'm a spare part.

• • •

The doctor estimated that Elle is just eight weeks pregnant, so I hoped I wouldn't have to think about the reality of being a dad for a while. Wrong. Today, a few short days after seeing the doctor, I have been wandering round a nightmarish shopping mall, looking blindly at prams, cots, baby gyms and other items too expensive to mention.

Shopping is never my idea of fun, but there was something different about the place today, something really creepy. I saw families everywhere – toddlers wandering aimlessly, babies screaming, little hands pulling at trouser-legs, pleading for the ice cream or the toy. There seemed to be kids all over the shop.

I can't believe how much stuff children need – parents were laden like pack horses with rucksacks, pushchairs were loaded with suspicious sacks of utensils and other shit. How did any of these people expect to actually cram any shopping into their cars?

It didn't take long to find out the answer – they didn't buy anything. They walked around, occasionally stopping to reach under the buggy for a camping stool or tyre lever, then wandered on. Sure, they might pick up a paper, or a new pair of bootees, but in reality this was just a day out. Shit. Is this what fatherhood makes of you? If so, I'm stuck in a nightmare.

We haven't even started to add up the cost of having a child and I wandered around endless displays of equipment. This was a complete contrast to just a few days ago, when the news seemed so incredible, and our lives were so special. In this mall we were surrounded by other couples, some just looking, like us, and some actually buying the stuff for their nursery. Women puffed and swore, their hands on the small of their backs as babies shifted. Men kept their heads down and tried to look interested.

We stuck at it for a while, prodding and poking at buggies and travel systems, mentally working out a rough total of pre-birth spending. But we didn't last long. I couldn't avoid feeling that my special experience has been taken over by an industry that chews up naive parents-to-be and spits them out minus their money. There are fathers-to-be everywhere and I am just another statistic waiting to be robbed of all my cash.

Big change

How much does a baby cost?

Back at the end of 2006, baby food manufacturer SMA carried out a ground-breaking survey of pre-birth spending by parents-to-be. They discovered that the average couple spent in excess of £1,500 on their baby before it was even born – while two per cent of those surveyed actually spent closer to £6,000. Though there's not been a comparable survey carried out since that time, you can be pretty sure that costs have increased and that you'll be looking at shelling out a couple of grand over the period between the positive pregnancy test and the birth. But what exactly do you need for a baby and what does it all cost? Let's take a closer look at what you should get in advance:

A pram. Possibly the most expensive single item you'll need to purchase, a pram is likely to set you back anything from £200-£500. You have a range of options, but generally the more flexible the pram is, the more expensive it is. Looking purely at cost is a bit of a false economy, some manufacturers have developed incredibly sophisticated 'travel systems' which comprise a pram, a pushchair and a car seat all in one. The advantage of these systems is they are extremely practical and adapt as your baby grows, the disadvantage is that they are bulky and cumbersome. A new travel system will set you back around £300.

Alternatively, you can take a shorter-term view and buy a more traditional pram which has a shorter usage span but provides more practical comfort. Once your baby is a bit older you can then move up to a pushchair. The advantage here is that you're using the right tools for each job, the disadvantage is that you'll have a house full of baby gadgets.

The most important consideration of all is 'what are you actually going to use it for?'. If you want to provide your baby with an extra daytime bed you might as well go for the ultra-traditional 'Silver Cross' style pram, but if you want something that will be used for serious off-road adventures, get something a bit more rugged. In any case, try before you buy – anything that can be folded one-handed is great, just in case you need to open or close it while holding a baby. And make sure it fits into the boot of your car. A pram or pushchair is something to seriously consider buying second hand. Most of them have such little use and the ones in charity shops or online are good for many more years. You can pick up a decent bargain for £30-£50.

A bed. Babies will sleep just about anywhere, but a bed is an essential item. Small babies are often happiest in a Moses basket or a carry cot as these feel a lot more secure than a larger crib. It's also a good idea to go for something that can be easily lifted and carried as you'll be lugging the baby around a fair bit over the first few weeks and months. You don't need a cot until the baby is about four to six months old. You can pick up a Moses basket and all the necessary bedding for about £50-£75.

Feeding facilities. If your partner is going to breastfeed this is an easy one. But if you're going along the route of formula milk, you'll need a steriliser and some bottles. You can get a steriliser that works in the microwave, and this is a great labour saver. When it comes to it, powdered milk is a much better bet than ready-made cartons and it works out a lot cheaper. Cost of all this is around £30-£50 depending on the brand.

Clothes. You'll need a set of clothes for the hospital – go for ones that are simple, cheap and easy to wash. One-piece romper suits are the best bet until your baby is about six months old. Clothes are one thing everyone else always buys you, so get them to buy short- and long-sleeved body suits, they're incredibly practical and useful. Don't buy designer clothes or your month-old baby will look like a chav. You should be able to buy all the essentials from a supermarket clothing line for about £50. Spending any more than that is pure vanity.

Car seat. If you're going to bring your baby home from hospital by car you have to have a properly fitted car seat. There are two types of seat available from birth, one for babies up to 10kg (around nine months) and one for babies up to 13kg (around 15 months). The first of these generally gives better support for smaller babies, though if your baby is really small, you'll probably need extra padding in the seat to keep it secure. You can swap to a bigger, forward facing seat at the 13kg milestone. Until your baby reaches that weight, you should put the seat so that it faces the rear of the car, and never put it on a front seat with an airbag.

Other good tips are to get the seat fitted by a decent store and learn how to fit it properly yourself – badly fitted seats have seriously affected performance. Try before you buy as not all seats fit all cars. And don't be tempted to buy a seat second-hand. If it's been damaged or in an accident it will be dangerous. Seats start from around £40-£50 and go up to around £150 or so.

NOTHING else. Apart from getting a few nappies in pre-birth and maybe a decent digital thermometer, you don't need anything else for the new arrival. Toys are a waste of time for the first six months, as is an expensively decorated nursery. The same goes for complete wastes of money such as baby baths, changing stations, multi-gyms and nappy bins. If relatives and friends are clamouring to buy stuff and they won't be put off, get them to give money instead – you'll be needing plenty of that once the prospect of childcare kicks in.

The true cost. In reality, if you shop around you should be able to get what you need for a shade under £250. Beg and borrow whatever you can – there's always someone trying to get rid of baby bits. Your tiny infant won't be image-conscious, so there's really no excuse to splurge. Wait until the little one is a bit older and buy something really useful then.

•   •   •

It is the start of week nine and Elle's appetite has dropped off so much that, as we both still cook for two, I am now beginning to show. Pretty soon I'll need a whole new wardrobe.

The things we eat are changing, too – out goes the fresh baked bread and the strong curries, the red wine and red meat. In comes bland chicken and fish and lots of fancy soft drinks made out of Elderflower and Ginseng and other compost heap crap.

None of this is to do with appetite, more with Elle's morning sickness, or more correctly her all day sickness. She doesn't have it too bad by all accounts – she's not actually throwing up – but she has a really strong reaction to some smells, including wine, and I'm trying to be supportive – so I'm easing off for a while. I yearn for a nice rare steak washed down with a couple of bottles of red, but I'm forcing myself to make do with sucking on a carrot and sipping flower juice. It does work for the sickness though, because I'm bloody sick of the whole thing. To be fair to Elle, she seems to miss those luxuries too – I hope this doesn't go on for the whole pregnancy.

Chapter Four
Dealing with problems

"For me the biggest single fear in the whole of our first pregnancy was not being in control. If anything went wrong I was powerless and that felt terrible." G, dad of two

---

What's happening?

Month four

Your partner's symptoms – your partner's body is adapting to the prospect of motherhood in two key ways – firstly her abdomen is changing shape to support the baby, so her waist will slowly disappear and clothes are going to be a lot tighter. Secondly, her skin may well be changing – most women find that their nipples and areolae (the ring of skin around the base of the nipple)become much darker and harder. It is also possible that a dark line develops down the middle of her belly. This mark is called a linea nigra and is a totally natural phenomenon that will fade after the birth. Some of the more unpleasant side-effects of early pregnancy will be easing now – particularly sickness and tiredness – so get ready for a serious burst of energy on her part.

Your baby – the baby's having a bit of a growth spurt too, as arms and legs will now be in proportion and hair will be growing on the little one's head. In fact hair will be growing just about everywhere as the baby is coated in a soft 'fur' called lanugo, which isn't a new model from Renault, it's a protective layer which, like the soft waxy coating on their skin called vernix, helps your baby cope with the fact that they are floating around in a giant sack of liquid.

I should have seen the warnings. Firstly, the weather this morning was as grey, chilly and uninviting as any Monday morning in history. I find it pretty hard to get up most days, but something about this morning was saying 'stay where you are'. Normally I need a few jabs in the ribs to wake me up and then a few flicks of the bedroom light to keep me awake. Even then, I drift off again until Elle returns from the bathroom and starts crashing around, getting dressed.

This morning I went back to sleep and woke a few minutes later to see Elle standing at the bedroom door. I sat straight up, because she was looking really worried.

"What?" I said.

"I don't know," she said, full of thought. "It's probably nothing, but…well I'm bleeding quite a bit."

Suddenly I was really awake. Even in a time of crisis I was keen to show off my new knowledge on pregnancy. A discharge of mucky brown blood is a fairly normal thing, fresh blood can mean danger. I've read the books, I could deal with this. "Fresh blood?" I asked.

"A little bit."

"Oh shit. Oh shit, oh shit."

OK, I couldn't deal with this. In fact I was crapping myself. We got dressed and went downstairs. I managed to make a cup of tea and she flicked through the baby books again, looking for something to put our minds at ease.

Though it made me feel really guilty to do so, I couldn't help thinking of the worst case, the idea that she might lose the baby. Elle has always been healthy – that must count for something?

Bollocks does it. All of the books I've read and all the people I've spoken to tell me the same thing – miscarriage is a hard, painful and unfair fact of life. The books offer a crumb of comfort that it is sometimes nature's way of ending a pregnancy that wasn't going to result in a healthy child, or one that might have harmed the mother. We're talking a very small crumb, here. All the experts agree that once the symptoms begin to show in detail, there is nothing to do except get into hospital and let fate take its course.

Facing a nightmare

The threat of miscarriage.

No one wants to think about miscarriage. I started out with the attitude that knowing all about it would somehow make the chance of it happening more real. If I shut it out, it couldn't happen to us. But that's total crap. You need to know the facts so, like it or not – and I know that you don't – here's some information on miscarriage from The Miscarriage Association, a support group helping people through this dreadful experience:

More than one in five pregnancies ends in miscarriage – around a quarter of a million in the UK each year.

Most miscarriages happen in the first three months of pregnancy – but they can happen up to the 24th week. Pregnancy loss after 24 weeks is known as stillbirth.

Any woman who is at risk of pregnancy is also at risk of miscarriage.

Most women never know what has caused them to miscarry. Investigations are generally limited to women who have had three or more miscarriages. Even after investigations, in many cases a specific cause is not found.

But:

Even after several miscarriages, most women have a good chance of a successful pregnancy.

Sex and miscarriage. You might be worried about poking around inside your partner at a time when the baby seems vulnerable, but the truth is that even if you're hung like a horse, sex isn't going to cause a miscarriage in early pregnancy. In fact, sex won't cause harm to the baby at any stage. But if your partner bleeds in early pregnancy, you might want to keep off the penetrative sex for a while, as it can be painful, stressful and not particularly sexy. There's plenty of other ways to get your oats, so get creative.

Elle went to the bathroom again, and returned with her eyes wet with tears. She was still bleeding. I went through the books, desperate to find something. But I wasn't going to find what I was looking for. The books couldn't tell me how to reassure her, or how to stop the sickness rising in my own gut. What they said, simply and correctly, was that I was helpless.

Elle was becoming increasingly upset. I tried to calm her by pointing out that she didn't have some of the symptoms. There were no cramps, no pains. Were there? By then anything was possible, she was feeling her worst fears. She was so scared, she didn't know what was symptom and what was imagination.

I felt completely useless. I had to take the initiative, so I suggested we call the doctors' surgery. There was no reply. We tried NHS Direct. A response, a return call and some comfort. But the nurse on the phone couldn't see Elle, or give any real advice from such a distance. She said we should contact the hospital.

That made it really scary. All of a sudden, we were in the middle of an emergency. We called the midwives' out of hours number and were given another number for the hospital's early pregnancy clinic. We called this and arranged to go straight in for a scan.

Hospitals for me have always been places for getting bad news. They are where people die, or are seriously ill. I couldn't link this place with anything positive. I smiled, I encouraged, I held Elle tight as we walked through the unfamiliar corridors, but I feared the worst.

By the time we reached the waiting room, my stomach was in knots. I had no idea how Elle was feeling, all I could see was her sad, blank face. A nurse spoke to us and left us with a form to fill. The NHS' reputation for pointless bureaucracy is unfair – this form was great therapy, I couldn't ever remember being so happy to focus on the dull details of name and address.

We sat for ages below a TV that was playing a chat show with the sound off, flicking pointlessly through old magazines, hugging each other and trying not to show each other how scared we were.

"Elle," a voice called, finally.

I was expecting another of those scenes that TV and film have turned to cliché. But the ultrasound room was a million miles from the huge, clinically white chamber of technology that American film producers can afford. It was small, dark and shabby with bright daylight shining around a curtain at the far end. It was more 'ooh-arr' than ER.

This was one anticlimax we didn't give a stuff about. We could have been sat on orange boxes as long as this scan worked out OK.

The ultrasound operator was no fun. She sighed impatiently as we confessed we hadn't read the information notice on the wall of the waiting room. No shit, lady, we had other things on our minds. Elle had to be sent off to empty her bladder before the internal scan could be attempted.

Eventually, we got started. It took a while to adjust my eyes to what I was seeing on the monitor. I didn't know whether I was looking for a problem or a baby. The screen showed something that looked like the inside of a football and right in the heart of it was a bean shaped blob. No, not a blob. A really clear, albeit tiny, baby. My baby. OK, our baby.

The operator clicked a few buttons and made some measurements, but said nothing. I began to worry that she hadn't spotted it, or even more worryingly, that I'd mistaken some essential organ for my kid.

I smiled and squeezed Elle's hand and she squeezed back, but she couldn't take her eyes off the screen. Eventually, after what felt like several hours, the operator spoke.

"So there's baby," she said. "Looking fine."

Fine. Oh yeah, right. Like this was just something she does every day. Well, OK, so it is. But the matter-of-fact attitude, the certainty of her description clashed so heavily with our fear of a few minutes earlier.

"But, but the bleeding…?" I stammered.

"Doesn't look like anything to worry about, I'll get doctor to speak to you," she replied. "Congratulations," she said, but not as if she meant it.

And we were out in the waiting room again, blinking in

the light, trying to take in what we had just seen as we were sent to another area to wait for the doctor. Eventually he poked his head around the door. "How are you doing?" he asked.

"Fine," we lied.

"Great, I'm a bit tied up, but I'll make sure someone comes and sees you soon," he said. His head disappeared, then returned. "You do know it's good news, right?" he asked.

For some reason we nodded. Actually no, we didn't know it was good news. They seemed to think we were looking to confirm the pregnancy, but we wanted to know the cause of the bleeding. In their hurry to give us what they thought we wanted, they'd missed the real issue.

A Sister arrived and finally put our minds at rest. No, the bleeding wasn't strictly 'normal' but it sometimes happened around this time. She said that some women bleed a little all the way through. Shit, I couldn't face one more morning like the one we've been through, let alone a few months' worth.

In the end, though, I feel reassured. The scan showed no problems. And I have seen our child for the first time – a little jumping bean with stubby arms and legs. When she'd finished moaning, the ultrasound operator actually pointed out the heart beating.

As emotional roller coasters go, it doesn't get much more extreme. I am so relieved we've ended it on a high. But it has shown me exactly how under-prepared I am for the emotional side of this pregnancy.

Any bloke in the situation I've just been through wants to be able to come up with the answers to all the worst fears. But short of a few years' medical training and a home ultrasound machine, I'm not going to provide much in the way of real help.

What I can give her is emotional support. That isn't easy when you're every bit as scared as the person you love. The trick is to prepare what you're going to say in any emergency situation, to appear cool, calm and in control. I hadn't wanted to think about this situation, but I know I need to plan for the worst and hope for the best. Life will always plonk me somewhere in between.

Crisis management

Knowing the medical basics

You can't hope to provide all the answers, unless you're a specialist or a bullshitter, and no, you shouldn't beat yourself up over this fact. Being told about bloody discharges and plugs of mucus isn't necessarily every man's cup of tea. Do you have to know about every one of your partner's bodily functions? I should damn well hope not. The symptoms of pregnancy can be graphic and disgusting. You don't need to explore them all to show your commitment.

But it's a good idea to know what can go wrong so you can offer support when it really counts. Here's a brief guide to the main problems that may (but hopefully won't) lie ahead:

Ectopic pregnancy. An ectopic pregnancy is one that takes place outside the uterus – normally in one of the fallopian tubes (which deliver the eggs from the ovaries to the uterus). This type of pregnancy is dangerous as the embryo has no space to develop and this can lead to serious problems, even to a burst tube. Most of the early signs of ectopic pregnancy are identical to normal pregnancy, but if at any time over the first four to ten weeks or so, your partner experiences serious pains in the abdomen, shoulder pain or bleeding from the vagina, coupled with nausea or dizziness, get her checked out as soon as possible.

Gestational diabetes. This condition is not like normal diabetes, as it will disappear after the birth, but it may also cause complications for the baby if it is unchecked. Women at risk of gestational diabetes include those who are older, more overweight, or who have a family history of diabetes. It's normally managed by making changes to the diet, but in extreme cases may have to involve insulin being given to the woman.

Pre-eclampsia. This is another sneaky condition, which is potentially life-threatening for your partner and the baby. The main problem is that the chief symptoms of pre-eclampsia are actually the same as a range of common, harmless pregnancy symptoms – like swelling and higher than usual blood pressure. If these symptoms all happen together, it needs checking out, as later stage pre-eclampsia can be extremely serious. If the condition is identified early enough, however, it can easily be monitored and controlled.

Pelvic pain. Late in pregnancy, Elle developed a pelvic problem that seriously limited her mobility and which was thought to have been a form of SPD – not the German political party, but symphysis pubis dysfunction, a disorder affecting the pubic bone in pregnancy. It limits mobility and can cause real pain prior to labour. For some people, it can even lead to lasting damage. We met midwives who knew about the disorder and were sympathetic, and we met other, normally more

senior, staff who basically said that it was all in the mind. If your partner is getting a lot of pain or discomfort in the pubic area around now,
there's a support group for the disorder and plenty of information on
the internet (try **www.nctpregnancyandbabycare.com**. It is also a
good idea to make sure your partner is able to consult an obstetric
physiotherapist, who can provide expert help to ensure your partner
minimises the impact on her physical well-being before, during and
after labour.

·   ·   ·

The scare worried us both. The excitement of seeing the
baby at nine weeks should have been massive, but instead
we have become really cautious. The problem with that, of
course, is that by being cautious we're constantly reminded of the idea of miscarriage. That's a big burden.

Not looking at clothes or toys, not telling any more people about the pregnancy, not buying anything for the
baby, not having sex because of the likelihood of more
bleeds, all this says that we fear losing the baby. It would
be better to be endlessly optimistic. But then what is sen-
sible and what is human can be worlds apart.

I know I'm making the situation worse by worrying all the time. Whenever Elle comes back from the bathroom I always ask if she's alright. I'm treating her as if she's desperately ill, as if the scan has given us reason to worry, rather than be comforted. I've started putting off decisions, wanting to leave them until we get to the 12 week mark, when the risk of miscarriage is reduced. I see it as some kind of secure barrier that will make me feel so much better in myself. I can't wait for it to arrive.

· · ·

Perhaps the best way to avoid worrying about miscarriage is to get wrapped up in other things. Week 11 has arrived, and that means a visit to the midwife for Elle's booking-in appointment.

The midwife is the number one cliché in my mind. I talked to my parents about what they went through and this has convinced me that midwives are always fierce, never sympathetic and all ancient. I already have a mental image of some kind of fire-breathing, starched uniform wearing octogenarian who treats any father-to-be attending an appointment as if he's a worthless, communist layabout.

After meeting her, I'd like to say that I was absolutely right on all counts. But the midwife is none of the above. She is close to retirement age, but that has only given me more faith in her experience.

She didn't seem to view me with suspicion. In fact, she barely viewed me at all in the appointment, focusing her attention on Elle. This is something I understand and even expect, but I don't like it. There would be a huge fuss if all mothers-to-be got treated the same. But it seems that fathers can take what they get and be grateful. I was allowed to ask a few questions and occasionally I got answers as well. But generally I was left with the feeling that I was taking up valuable chair space.

It isn't the first – and I'm sure it won't be the last – time that spare part feeling surfaces in this pregnancy. I want to be there for every push and prod, every puff and blow. The only other person who has a similar commitment to stick by Elle is the midwife, and this one doesn't seem to welcome my involvement. So we are rivals, enemies. This is a battle of wills I am determined to win.

The more I was sidelined by the midwife, the more I cut in, the less my opinion was asked for, the more it was given. Poor Elle must have felt like the net judge at Wimbledon, mediating a rally between us. By the end of the appointment I felt as if I'd established a firm position. This woman might not remember my name, but she knows I am serious. Or at least seriously odd.

Elle gave me a strange look as we walked to the car. I asked her what was wrong. "You're so funny, asking all those questions," she said. I don't think she minds but it would be pushing it to say she's impressed. I think she's surprised and probably a bit amused. I hope she's comforted, I take an interest because I want to get involved, but also because I want her to know that I'm fighting for her. I guess it comes back to feeling so powerless in the scan room.

Not seen and not heard

Trying to deal with the midwife

Good, bad or just ugly, the midwife is the closest thing you will have to a guide in pregnancy, and though your partner may well rely on her, you might end up feeling edged out. It's your job to change that; she will just do what she always does – and that means she'll focus entirely on your partner's needs.

As the appointments generally involved blood pressure monitoring and, later, heartbeat checks etc, Elle was often focused on being prodded and poked and forgot to ask any questions we wanted answered. So I'd make sure we talked about it first, then asked those questions myself.

Once you've established eye contact with a midwife, you can then start to work on a relationship. Ten, 11, 12 months later, our midwife still didn't know my name, or what I did for a living, but she respected my right to be there.

The most exciting result of this appointment was the huge folder of leaflets, books and other stuff that Elle has been given. We took them home and laughed at the efforts rival baby product firms make to get their hands on our cash.

One of the most pathetic is a book called 'Emma's Diary' in which Emma details her experiences along with those of her friends from a broad ethnic, cultural and class background. It's terrible. Some effort has been put in to offer a wide range of experience, but it's written with such a clear agenda – the poor friend with a bun in the oven and no ring on her finger faces endless disasters, while Tom and Katy Middle-Class (not their real names) take a couple of hours out from their busy middle management lives to have a baby whose shit doesn't stink. I pity poor Emma for having friends like these, but my real sympathy is for the millions of mothers-to-be who are expected to read this bollocks.

Much more interesting was the bundle of vouchers giving us a variety of free samples, gift packs and other goodies which mean we can hit the shops again. So now, at the end of the day, we have a couple of carrier bags full of stuff. I need to do a bit more research to work out what the hell half the things we've been given are used for. But it's a relief to know that we now have all the nipple cream we can eat.

•   •   •

The 12 week landmark has sneaked up on us. It's changed nothing, I am still worried about the idea of making fixed plans and we are both still scared by the occasional bleeds that Elle is having.

Twelve weeks does mark something, however. After our crap efforts to tell our families about our good news, we have decided to break the good news to friends and colleagues.

This isn't going to be easy, either. Families can learn how

to be tactful over the years. Because they love you, they are good at sounding pleased at any good news you have to offer. The same is partly true for friends – good friends anyway – but colleagues aren't required to be delighted for you. I can't help but feel that the reality of life post-baby is about to kick in.

Elle has it the hardest. Working in business, she faces lots of prejudice from day to day anyway. Now she's got to cope with men saying 'I wondered when that was going to happen' when she breaks the news, as if pregnancy was some kind of character flaw. Many of them will assume unfairly that this is the end of her working life.

Colleagues aren't such a problem when you work for yourself like I do, but I'm still nervous about telling my friends. I guess I'm worried about losing my youth and independence, especially as we're planning for me to take on the lion's share of looking after the kid with Elle going back to work part time.

I can just imagine what my mates will say about me becoming that dreaded thing 'the househusband'. Actually, they probably won't give a toss, most of them think I spend my days sitting in front of the TV as it is.

Richard and Judy and you?

Being a stay at home dad

It's true that birth is actually a life changing experience – so it's also the perfect chance to change a few other areas of life too. It's why so many people move house with a baby on the way. A survey of new fathers showed that more than 40 per cent want to stay at home with the baby. Yet only a few actually go on to do that. Why?

There's a few reasons – partly social, partly financial. The man is still seen as the main wage earner, the woman as the best carer. But the world is shifting, and the community of stay at home dads is getting stronger all the time. Support networks and online communities are there to help men cope with some of the crap they encounter when making this decision for themselves.

It's a tough issue, and one that is looked at in detail in Richard Hallows' Full Time Father (White Ladder), but the basic pros and cons are pretty clear. If you don't mind your own company and you're happy watching daytime TV while ironing baby clothes or cleaning up milk vomit then you've got what it takes. If you want an incredible chance to bond with your child and discover your own resourcefulness, then you really should consider it.

In fact, what worries me more is the fear that I'll give up being my old self after this kid arrives. I want to be reassured by the strength of my own convictions – the belief that I will somehow succeed in juggling my work and childcare in spite of the obvious strain it'll put on my time management skills.

Rather than waste time contacting everyone, I simply broke the news to an old journalism colleague of mine. Sure enough the gossip spread like wildfire. Within hours of our boozy lunch, half a dozen friends got in touch to check, partly tongue in cheek, whether this new arrival would be the end of my 'career' ambitions. Right now it's hard to believe that it isn't.

Chapter Five
Emotional changes

"I found I wasn't so interested in sex, not because my wife wasn't beautiful, but because I saw her as the 'mothership' for our child." P, dad of one.

What's happening?

Month five

Your partner's symptoms – The increased weight of the growing baby may start to show itself in other areas. Your partner will start to be a bit breathless if she's having to spend any sustained period standing, and she may get more stitches and rib pains than before. She will also sweat more profusely and will notice other side-effects like bleeding gums and a blocked nose.

Your baby — now that your baby has inner ears, tastebuds and a functioning respiratory system, there's a lot more stimuli for the little soul and a lot more activity as a result. Sudden loud noises or music can startle the baby even at this early stage.

While I've been worrying about the future, Elle's been getting on with the present. The sickness has eased and her appetite's coming back slowly, but she still reacts to some smells and tastes. By far the worst symptom is tiredness. She gets through the day with just enough energy to make it home. Her evenings are short and quiet, her nights long and uncomfortable.

Tiredness is common, but normally from about 14 weeks things start to become a little easier, and it's when most women get back some of their zest for life. It's a landmark I can't wait to see for one particular, selfish reason. Elle has always needed her full eight hours' sleep, but she is starting to drag herself off to bed at nine. We aren't seeing much of each other. In other words, I'm starting to fret about sex.

I'm not one of those men who wants a shag every Saturday night in the gap between Casualty and Match of the Day.

But it's been a couple of weeks now, and I'm starting to think about the idea of going without in the longer term.

I don't want to use the old gag about sex being all ups and downs, but it is a bit of a feast followed by famine. Not that I'm being starved; if anything I'm the one holding back. To be honest, I haven't worked out how to handle sex in this pregnancy. Do I assume things will carry on as normal? Do I change my attitude about what is expected of me in bed? Or do I give myself a helping hand in the good old spirit of Do It Yourself?

The answer, of course, is all of the above. I'm only going to get through this most personal part of the process by keeping my own basic needs under control, trying to find out what Elle is happy and comfortable with and learning to cope with a lower position in the pecker, sorry, pecking order than before. I mean, sod it, it's only short term. Isn't it?

Get it on

Sex in pregnancy (part one)

Sex is what got you here in the first place, so you ought to be an expert in the subject by now, yeah? Not a bit of it. Pregnant sex is a whole new ball game, with its own rules, some of which are great for you, and others which are frankly odd. Here's a guide to the whole new ball game:

Breasts. Those tits are bigger, fuller and more sensitive than ever before. If you ever wondered what she'd look like with a boob job you're about to find out, and the best thing is that you've not had to shell out £3,000 for the privilege. These fulsome funbags certainly seem like a major perk for you when they're compared with most other symptoms of pregnancy, but before you begin your blissful ascent of the north face of her breasts, remember also that they are likely to be sore – later in pregnancy they may become full of milk and that can be really painful, as well as messy when they have the odd leak at times of high stimulation. So by all means explore the new and strange landscape of your partner, but treat it with respect, rather than sticking your flagpole in the first crevice you find.

An interesting position. Positions in the early days are less of an issue than when there's a giant bump in the way (see sex part two, chapter eight), but you may still want to keep things more gentle and give up a little bit of the control in the bedroom. If you let your partner 'ride' you, she can control the depth of the penetration and the vigour of the sex. Positions to avoid throughout pregnancy, unless your partner is very keen, include doggy style and anything that involves hanging from the ceiling. The former leads to very deep penetration that she may find uncomfortable, the latter is just plain wrong.

As with the breasts, there's an advisory warning attached to all penetrative sex in pregnancy – let your partner decide how lively things should get, otherwise be gentle. If all is going well with the pregnancy, there's no risk to the baby at all, but if there's any bleeding or if her doctor tells her to ease off for a while, respect that and back off.

Risk-free sex. Another major advantage of sex in pregnancy might seem an obvious one, but it can be really liberating to know you can't get her pregnant. Free of the constraints of contraception, you might find you're actually having the most spontaneous, exciting sex of your life. Don't be surprised if she wants to make love all over the house, it's an extremely liberating time. Many women find that, once they are over the initial period of nausea and sickness and into the 'blooming' phase, sex becomes incredibly pleasurable. Those swollen breasts and an increasingly sensitive vagina and clitoris can combine to create the most mind-blowing sex – hell, she might even start to enjoy it too.

Ups and downs. There's a flipside of course, and that comes when you're both completely out of synch with regard to sex drive. Some men go off sex altogether, either out of a fear that they'll harm the baby or because they share the feelings of our surveyed dad at the start of this chapter, who wanted to refrain from sex out of respect. In some situations this can misfire badly, especially if you aren't communicating your love and support to your partner in other, equally loving ways. It's not unheard of for a woman to get a really strong sex drive in pregnancy, and if you're standing back while she's on heat, there's going to be one almighty row.

Satisfaction action. Finding other ways to satisfy each other when one or other of you doesn't fancy penetrative sex can be tough. Giving oral sex isn't always easy for men in pregnancy: some women have strong smelling discharges that can be pretty off-putting, while expecting her to go down on you all the time might be a bit harsh, considering how hard it is for her to suppress the gag instinct at the best of times. It might be a good time to read that sensual massage book and try out a few new moves. Just touching, stroking and mutually masturbating can keep the intimacy that you both need.

Pleasing yourself. If you do find yourself going through a bit of a dry spell, you do always have the option of helping yourself. People don't talk much about masturbation – it's still regarded by some as a sin and by others as something dirty or shameful. This is very bad news for most dads-to-be, who will either have to learn extreme self-control or the ability to have a quick one off the wrist without feeling like a naughty schoolboy who's going straight to hell. Having a quick wank can ease all those feelings of frustration and resentment that otherwise might spill over into something serious. Most blokes I know actually masturbate well beyond their teenage years, though only a few of them are open and honest about it, which is a real shame. I'm not saying it's something to bring up at a board meeting, but it is a very useful, safe and totally free weapon in your war against sexual frustration. So use it. But don't wear it out.

One thing I know for sure, doing without sex is better than bothering her all the time. She has started having little mood swings, which add to the sickness and tiredness and mean she's not exactly attached to my private parts at present. I would like to stay attached to them, so I'll keep quiet for a bit.

"Where did I leave those scissors?"

Coping with mood swings

If you thought that hormones just do strange physical things to your partner, you should try watching a soppy film with her. Elle would cry buckets at a slightly gloomy weather report and would howl with sympathy whenever Tom failed to catch Jerry. OK, that's a bit of an exaggeration, but her moods did begin to swing, albeit gently, with a fair degree of regularity.

Few women are really moody during pregnancy, their emotions – like their senses – are often just heightened. So the old cliché about pregnant women flying off the handle at the slightest thing is mainly pub banter. If you behave as you normally would, but with a bit more sensitivity, you'll probably avoid too much hassle. So don't forget birthdays, anniversaries and special occasions, don't make more work for your partner around the house, don't tell her you're thinking of giving up work and driving round Europe on a Harley.

Try to think of her moodiness as a symptom of pregnancy, rather like morning sickness. When she started throwing up or feeling ill, your first thought wasn't 'oh no, she's going to be like this every day for the rest of our lives,' was it? So if she snaps a bit now and then, smile, apologise and put it down to the miracle of birth. Making a big issue out of it won't solve anything, and you'll have to back down anyway. So be wise, take a deep breath and this too shall pass.

• • •

On the subject of profiles, until now Elle's parents have been keeping theirs high, keen to show that they are interested, informed and in my face. They call all the time with advice on a variety of subjects, mainly diet and exercise. Had the advice been invited, it would be welcome, but I know that their ideas on childcare belong with Spangles and Tartan trousers in the mid-Seventies.

I also know that they mean well, but I take their comments as seriously as that of my Nan, who campaigns for Guinness to be available on prescription. According to her, a bottle a day is Elle's answer. It would take at least that for her to be able to cope with the quick-fire questioning of her parents.

The worst part – and they are not the only relations or friends guilty of this – is that although I'm happy to deal with all their questions, they don't seem to believe I could possibly know anything about the pregnancy. It is very patronising, and it makes me feel like shit. Months before antenatal classes, I'm getting lots of early practice at deep breathing techniques.

"And another thing…"

Dealing with unwanted opinions

Pregnancy can make you feel a bit like you're under attack, even if everything's going smoothly. If your partner is having a rough time of it, there will be a million different opinions blasting at her from relatives and well-wishers. Your job is intervention and information manage-ment. Help her sort the good intentions from the crap, and then keep the crap at bay. There's nothing more upsetting than some dried up old spinster of a great aunt going on about how eating apples in pregnan-cy causes typhoid.

So don't be afraid to act tough. Setting the boundaries of acceptable behaviour now means that when the baby is born people will respect your privacy that much more. Right now you're probably being patron-ised by mothers who think they know better, and bizarrely by fathers as well, but don't let them wind you up – this is your show and you can run it any way that makes you and your partner comfortable.

My parents don't bombard us with questions, but they have done something that threw me right off track. They came over for lunch yesterday – Mothers' Day – and brought Elle a present. It was so strange, I couldn't get my head around the idea that she is going to be a mother. It sounds so grown-up. We will be parents, I will be a father, and soon. None of this should come as much of a surprise to me, but I hadn't put it in context, I'm so wrapped up in the idea of the pregnancy that I haven't thought much about the end product. It's also weird that this revelation should come from my parents – suddenly we are going to be equals, all parents together. It feels like a massive and sudden leap into some kind of secret society and I don't know if I'm comfortable with it.

• • •

Because of the emergency scan after nine weeks, the hospital decided not to do a 12 week scan. We talked this over with the midwife and she agreed that we should get a scan done after all. Actually she said something like 'this is your baby and you need to get what you can. Be selfish, put yourselves first'. This isn't great advice, too much of that sort of crap just screws everything up for everyone. But we've already sussed that in the harsh world of free health-care, those who keep silent are dumb. Anyhow, we don't want the Earth, just the chance to take another look at that jumping bean.

So today we were back in the hospital, in the same area where we'd sat and imagined the worst. This time we were totally different people, we followed the instructions carefully, beamed at the moody attendants and sat quietly as the operator made sense of the shadows and patterns on the screen. It was quite frustrating to watch the scan, which was of the traditional, gel on the belly type. It was fuzzier and less clear than the internal nine week job.

The operator was pointing out the baby lying at the bottom of the screen when suddenly it gave a huge jump, shot into the centre of the shot, did a backflip and waved at us. OK, so I made up those last two, but it definitely jumped, a massive leap that was captured for ever, as the operator printed off a photo for us to keep.

The picture is a big bonus. The people in the ultrasound unit recommended that we shouldn't try to get pictures until 20 weeks, but this gives us something real to hang on to. I don't care that my child now looks like a misshapen monkey nut, I love it, and, as long as it doesn't actually stay like that, I know I'll look back with great affection on this early snapshot.

Elle feels the same, only more so. When we got back from the hospital, she raced to the scanner and computer and produced a range of copies, enlargements, reductions, T-shirts and posters. If a mother's love for her child can be measured out in ink and paper, then our baby has a bright future. We now have more pictures of our 12 week old foetus than we do of each other after eight years together.

The measurements taken by the ultrasound operator match the due date calculated at the doctor's, meaning that our child was almost certainly conceived during our drunken anniversary celebration. I feel a bit guilty at the thought of a new life springing from so much alcohol, but at least it was a happy start to life.

•   •   •

The pace of life in general seems to have taken over, the only signs of the pregnancy are baby magazines and clothes catalogues littering our lounge. And I mean littering. Elle's general tiredness keeps her from doing much around the house and I'm worried that if I start doing the housework I'll get the job permanently.

I don't want to sell myself short here, there are things I'm good at – washing up is one of my key skills. I can also vacuum pretty well. But I'm like a high class cleaning prostitute, I have boundaries. I don't dust, I don't iron, I don't do French. No aprons.

And yet, some of this stuff simply has to be done. Washing, for example, is now a grey area, as is cooking. Both seem to be important, but does that mean I have to take the initiative? Probably. If you weigh up the pros and cons, all I have on my side is the fact that I'm crap at these things, while Elle has all the emotional strings, like needing a good diet and clean clothes for work. I feel abused, but I don't think there's much point in complaining.

"How long do you boil lettuce?"
Your role as hired slave

It sometimes feels that the moment you learned your partner was pregnant you agreed to become her hired slave. And up to a point that's true – there are many things that she'll be unable or unwilling to do in her state that must be picked up by other people and easing the pressure of chores and such like is probably your largest responsibility this side of labour. But that doesn't mean you have to do it all – it might mean managing a team of willing and non-judgmental relatives to help with ironing, cooking, cleaning etc. If you can afford it, you could also consider getting some paid help – it won't be for long, and sending out your ironing instead of sweating over it all evening is well worth the price of a takeaway.

Cooking is a real problem, made worse by the fact that it has become a battle of wills. Elle's appetite is still poor, and she would skip meals if it was left to her – but I keep pushing her, offering a banana here, a cheese sandwich there. I struggle to find new ways to present boiled vegetables, and with summer coming I know I'll be just as limp with salad.

A few days ago I thought I had it cracked, thanks to my new friend the dried apricot. According to food experts, this wrinkled piece of rubbery gunk is the answer to all our prayers. One small portion boosts Elle's diet and saves me from being creative. This flawless plan – involving a quick trip to the supermarket where I cleared the shelf of dried apricots – fell apart when Elle got sick of the damned fruit after the first bag.

·   ·   ·

Fortunately, as so often happens in life, fate has saved me from making an even bigger arse of myself. Elle's zest has returned. Well, maybe 'zest' is pushing it a bit – she's still tired all the time – but she's taken over in the kitchen again. Apricots are banned.

In my rediscovered free time, I've written a feature for a website on the first few weeks of Elle's pregnancy. It's short, and I thought it was just a bit of fun but it has produced a couple of big reactions which stopped me in my tracks.

The first has come from an old boss of mine, a proud and devoted mother. I told her about the feature and she promised to take a look. When I saw her next, she gave me a dark look and shook her head.

"I'm angry with you," she said. "I can't believe you can say this," she added, jabbing at a copy of the feature. She pointed out the section that had upset her, in which I said I 'feel like a louse for inflicting months of discomfort and disruption on someone I love so much'.

She said that no mother would feel that something as special as a baby was a 'disruption'. She might be right. But I was talking about me. Me. It may not have been how the 'burden' of pregnancy is viewed by Elle, or by any mother, but it is absolutely true for me. When she saw the baby on the monitor at the hospital for the first time, I'm sure she felt real elation – it probably even made up for the nausea and tiredness. But I haven't got that attachment, the immediate feeling that you can only get when something inside you is depending on you for its existence. All I have is love for my wife, and a desire to keep her and the baby secure. If I want to feel like a louse, I'm damned if anyone's going to stop me, because I want to be part of the relationship that is bonding between my wife and our child.

The second response was from a friend in business. His family means everything to him, though he is separated and rarely sees his children.

"I can't believe you've missed the more important part," he spluttered.

I shrugged, lost for words. I couldn't imagine what it was I'd forgotten.

"No mention of the pressure to earn money to support the family?" he said, staring in amazement at me, expecting the answer to hit me like a wet fish.

"I suppose," I said.

"No suppose about it," he snapped. "It's the single biggest pressure. I used to lie awake at night wondering what would happen if I lost my job. I mean, I used to worry before – but as soon as she was pregnant it all got much more serious." He stopped and thought for a few moments. "But then you just don't have that, do you?"

I smiled, shrugged and changed the subject. But now my mind keeps returning to his comments. Maybe he is right. As Elle is the main wage earner, I haven't needed to think too much about it. But in a few months she's going on maternity leave and things are going to get tight. And I haven't even started to think about what happens afterwards.

We've planned things quite well and have a few savings, but any little disaster could throw all that off. We've both been through a fair share of upheaval in our working lives – company closures, redundancies, shit bosses, crap conditions – but we've always come through. Perhaps I just have faith in our ability to make something out of the situation. Perhaps I just haven't given it enough thought. Maybe I do have something to panic about after all.

I've tried to think of friends in similar situations. One of my former colleagues is a single father – he's juggled his full time job with childcare. He's used a nursery and that isn't what we want. So if I do have to start bringing in a more reliable income, it needs to be part time at best.

Another friend runs a business from home, supporting his wife and three children. He is a success story, a man in complete control of his finances and his relationships. He has the flexibility to adapt to any situation and the money to raise his family.

I liked the sound of this, so I talked to him about the realities of his situation. Sure, he agreed, he has a good balance, and he's rarely short of work. But this is the result of 10 years' hard graft. He told me about the early days, the long hours, the lack of sleep, not taking a holiday for fear of losing work. All the usual pressures that go with starting a business – intensified by the pressure of knowing that you have a child on the way. But, he conceded, life is good now. It has been worth it.

So by the sounds of it I should be in flexible, part time work with a high guaranteed income. But what to choose? Politics, dentistry or royalty? No, all the jobs with large salaries and short hours have been taken.

A return to 'proper' full time work wouldn't ease any worries, except those of our parents, who belong to a generation that wrongly believes the words Status Quo stand for both quality of music and quality of life. We will only be happy if we live life in a way that we can honestly call our own. Money worries are a fact of all our lives, whether we're in control of the purse strings or not. I might not feel the same level of pressure as my breadwinning friend, but that doesn't mean I don't want the best for my family. I'll do what it takes to keep our financial future secure, but I'm not about to start panicking about things I can't control.

Chapter Six
The medical side

"I wanted to be there for all the new things – scans and all the rest. I don't think I helped much, but no-one was going to keep me away." B, dad of one.

What's happening?

Month six

Your partner's symptoms – your partner will be able to feel the baby kicking on a regular basis around now – and so should you. This is great news as it is the first time you've been able to interact with the baby. Your partner will be feeling increasingly tired and will also be struggling to sleep – which all adds up to the prospect of some bad moods. She may well be having even more digestive problems – particularly heartburn – which won't be adding to the feeling of goodwill.

Your baby – By the end of this month your baby is fully formed and may stand a fair chance of surviving outside of the uterus if born prematurely. But the next three months are all important for your baby's development and growth. Even though it seems as if you're both just hanging around, waiting for the baby to arrive, encourage your partner to keep eating healthily and exercising regularly.

Life has started to speed up worryingly. Weeks are zipping past so quickly that another big milestone has passed us by.

During the booking in appointment, the midwife talked about a routine, optional blood test for disorders like Spina Bifida and Down's Syndrome at 15 weeks. We'd both shaken our heads at the idea and the suggestion that it carried with it and I forgot all about it.

But now that milestone is long gone, we have been reminded, by books rather than the midwife, that this option had been available. I asked Elle how she felt about missing it.

Unlike me, she has been giving it some serious thought. It's understandable – the responsibility of caring for a disabled child falls on both parents, but if a couple decide to abort a foetus, suddenly the balance swings towards the mother. She has to deny her instincts and agree to abort something that she has already started to bond with.

I'm not saying I understand the moral reasons for or against abortion, but I know that if it is necessary, for medical or social reasons, it could never be seen as an easy option.

For Elle, it isn't an option. Which for me is a big relief, because I want us to care for our child whatever. We've both stayed as opposed to testing as we were on that first midwife appointment. I'd say that the decision isn't the important thing, the unity is.

The toughest test

Testing and scanning for problems

The low down. Testing for abnormalities and disabilities is a pretty tough issue, and it's one that you have to get your head around. If your partner is over 35 there is a strong chance that some form of testing may be recommended as the chance of congenital defects are higher. Whether or not you feel comfortable making the final decision to test or not, you have a right to know the facts of the situation. This is a short guide to what's available and what it all means:

Screening. There are two types of test – screening tests and diagnostic tests. A screening test can give you an idea of the likelihood of your child developing a serious developmental disorder like Spina Bifida or a chromosomal disorder like Down's Syndrome. Screening tests normally involve taking blood at around 15-16 weeks and testing it, although there is another type of screening test called a nuchal fold scan which also shows the likelihood of a particular condition. Neither of these tests are conclusive, but they can give some reassurance that the chances are slim. Results indicate the probability of your baby being born healthy – say one in 500 – which allows you to proceed with more confidence.

What's next? A more detailed form of testing is a diagnostic test. There are two main types of tes: amniocentesis, a test for Down's, Spina Bifida and other genetic abnormalities, which examines a small sample of amniotic fluid from around the baby, and CVS (chorionic villus sampling) which tests for Down's and other genetic abnormalities but not Spina Bifida. CVS takes a sample of tissue from the placenta. Both these tests carry a miniscule (less than one per cent) risk of miscarriage, but both are completely accurate. The advantage of CVS is that it is normally carried out at around 12 weeks, while amniocentesis is usually carried out around 18 weeks. If the test results showed a serious problem, CVS would allow a decision to be taken on termination at an earlier stage which would be safer for your partner.

So in a nutshell, the deeper you get into testing, the riskier it is, though it is more likely to prove conclusive. It's an area that needs specialist medical help, but that doesn't mean you should just listen to the doctor or midwife and ignore your own feelings. Testing isn't about a pregnancy, it's about a child, or even an adult, that you're going to have to help care for. You need to be informed so you can make the wisest choice.

The anatomy scan. While the 12 week dating scan is a formality (and in some regions of the UK it isn't even an option), the anatomy scan at 20 weeks is a bigger deal and takes a while to go through. It's an opportunity for the hospital to check up on issues like cleft lip and palate, Spina Bifida and any other deformities or abnormalities that couldn't be picked up at an earlier stage. Rather like the tests, it carries with it the possibility of a potentially heartbreaking decision over termination if there are serious problems.

Gender politics. For most people, however, the anatomy scan means just one thing – the chance to find out their baby's sex. Hospitals are finally getting the message across that guessing gender is a risky business. Just 10 per cent of the fathers surveyed tried to find out the baby's sex early. A couple of others actually thought the bonding issue went the other way: if they were secretly hoping for a boy and discovered early on that it was a girl, they'd worry about feeling a bit less attached to the baby.

It's obviously a personal issue, but if you are desperate to find out and don't want to get the brush off from a lawyer-shy hospital you could pay to have a private scan done at a slightly later stage than the traditional 20 week anatomy scan. You'd have a better chance of seeing the business end of the baby clearly and some private clinics have the latest technology which gives a much more realistic image (some even in colour and 3-D) than the fuzzy blobs on standard ultrasound kit. It'll cost you, but if you're one of those guys who just can't wait, it might be worth it. The official line on scans is that they are a medical procedure and should therefore only be used for medical reasons, not because you can't choose between My Little Pony and Thomas the Tank Engine wallpaper.

Moments like that are coming up throughout the pregnancy, small but crucial decisions that may have an impact for years afterwards. I think it is partly why so many men think fatherhood makes them grow up suddenly. The truth is, it doesn't make me feel any more adult, just more aware of the consequences of my actions. It makes me think and sometimes it scares me. Sometimes these decisions take a while to be reached, but I try never to avoid them. Well, almost never.

I've taken one decision that I've been putting off from day one. The more I've allowed myself to delay, the harder it has become. In the end I have decided simply to face it, even though I could put it off for many more weeks, months even.

Today, I convert the relaxing, crowded, creative haven formerly known as The Study into the soft, fluffy, book free chamber of horrors that is to become The Nursery.

I've worked alone, like a convict cracking rocks. I've bought a pile of cardboard crates, miniature coffins for my stuff, and filled them with most of the books, stationery and crap that I've collected over the years.

I am allowed just three bookshelves, moved to a new location in our bedroom, and a small desk. I have spent a stupid amount of time weighing up which books to take with me to this desert island, repeating the process for CDs, pens, paper and ornaments.

It is pathetic. I have agonised over ring binders and high-lighter pens, struggled to squeeze extra books onto my permitted shelving. Even worse than the rationing, working in the bedroom will mean keeping my desk tidy, filing and even, God forbid, throwing things away.

The fact that my little empire can be packed so easily into boxes to make way for the baby raises many questions over my future work. Is it a sign of things to come? Will any of these boxes see the light of day again, or will they just move from loft to dump without another thought. It makes me uneasy. How can I work without my stuff?

Elle has clearly entered the unsympathetic phase of pregnancy, pointing out that I have both pen and paper at my disposal, and that my laptop needs very little space as it can, apparently, be used on my lap. Yes, yes, very funny, but what about my cricket trophy, my hipflask and my hand held paper shredder?

Anyway, back to the decoration of the nursery. As it is replacing my study, I've been allowed a bit of freedom over the choice of décor. I've settled on cream for the walls, the door and the ceiling. The floorboards have survived, but they show many traces of the struggle. The overall effect is, well, cream. It is a blank canvas on which to stamp the individuality of our child. And it's used up all that old cream paint.

Now all we need is a clear idea of our child's sex and a big dose of inspiration to create a memorable and attractive room. Both are a long way off. For the time being it is set to stay as a big, off-white, empty shell. I stand in it and remember happy days. I need to get out more.

·   ·   ·

Three months ago I didn't even know the baby existed. Now it has its own bedroom, a wardrobe, a crib and a bath. It has a load of prospective babysitters and a whole street of interested well-wishers. And yet it still isn't even halfway to being born. Talk about attention seeking.

Every part of life seems to be about the baby right now. In the last couple of weeks we've had trips to the midwife for blood pressure checks and a quick listen to the baby's heartbeat, to the obstetrician for a consultation on the back problems that Elle has started to experience and to the doctor for another pointless session of chatting about the weather.

We've even taken on an allotment so that next year we can grow all the vegetables for the baby's food. There is a good point to this, it is somewhere we can go which doesn't have a baby magazine, a doctor's appointment card or a fluffy toy anywhere in sight. It is a small site, but it feels like an island, an oasis in the desert of antenatal care. We both get a bit stressed about the fact that babies are apparently the only subject on the minds of parents and family, even friends and colleagues. So it's good to have somewhere to slide off to.

Anyway, back to babies. Next week is the 19th of the pregnancy and Elle is booked for another session with our old friends in the ultrasound room. It'll be a full six weeks since we saw them and I just know they'll be dying to catch up with us.

This is the anatomy scan, the big one. This is the time when the operator checks for club feet, hare lips, heart and spine problems. All massive, life changing things. We're nervously awaiting confirmation of our baby's good health. But I can't get away from the fact that this is also the moment when we might get an idea of the baby's sex.

Does it really matter? Not particularly. It's possible that

the Giles bloodline would die out if we didn't produce a son, and that in turn might mean the sale and dispersal of our family heirlooms – though whether we'd get much more than a fiver for my Nan's hostess trolley and expanding globe cigarette holder remains to be seen.

I know my Nan would like a boy, I suspect my mother-in-law would like a girl. Elle is undecided. I'd just like a baby, though of course I'll reserve the right to send it back if it starts supporting Man United.

There's no point in knowing the baby's gender for financial or practical reasons. Who cares if we have to wait to paint that pink or blue mural on the cream study, sorry nursery, wall. The same goes for clothes – white and pastel shades will do just fine for the first few months.

For my money, the only real reason for knowing the baby's sex at this stage is to start bonding. For the last three months we've referred to our baby as 'the blob', which is all well and true to photographic evidence. But nothing stops you bonding quite like the feeling you're having a child that looks like something from a 1950s disaster movie.

Guessing means nothing as I've also been warned how difficult it is to get information about gender from the ultrasound operator. In our age of law suits, hospitals have to be extra careful about telling future parents such things. It's easy to make mistakes, and apart from the inconvenience of getting it wrong, there's a real risk of throwing off that bond between child and parents if they don't get what they expect.

So maybe we shouldn't ask. But then, it would be good to know. But then, they won't tell us, so then…bugger it, we'll see.

• • •

Or not. Another bad day at the ultrasound as our baby again refused to behave itself. Everything started so well, I found a parking space in the same county as the hospital, walked just half a mile to the department and waited for no longer than the time it takes to Improve Your Word Power in a four year old copy of Reader's Digest.

But as soon as we were in and the monitor was switched on, the baby resisted all attempts to measure, monitor and watch its behaviour. A fair amount of poking and pushing later and the only result was that Elle's bladder was in serious danger of exploding.

The ultrasound operator gave up in the end, deciding that we need to come back when the baby's in a better position, when it is bigger and when the newer, more powerful ultrasound machine is available.

It's a big anticlimax. Everything about this scan was important to us, and we feel let down by the lack of a result. After all the fuss over whether we would ask about the gender, I didn't even think to mention it.

•   •   •

Elle is now at the halfway stage. In about 20 weeks we will have a baby, a new life, and I will be its father. It's a thought that is both exciting and petrifying. And I am not at all ready for it. If I'm going to do the slightest justice to my child, I have to pull myself together now. Time is running out. We've been to stay with my parents for a week – our last holiday before the baby – and that strange feeling I had on Mothers' Day reappeared. I've never known them talk so much about their own experiences, I've found out loads of stuff about my childhood that I didn't know, but even more about what my parents were like at our age. It explains a lot and it's one of the most unexpected and surprising bits of the pregnancy so far.

Meanwhile, it's back to the ultrasound room. We've got back from holiday to find the appointment letter for the rescan, set for the middle of next week, just a fortnight after the disappointing first effort.

All the hopes and fears from that first scan are back. The gender issue has slipped a bit on the order of priorities, the bigger concern now is that everything is where it should be.

•   •   •

This time the baby was in a better mood and a clearer position. We had a great view of perfect fast bowler's hands and footballer's feet. We even saw the little valves of the heart at work. Everything else seemed to check out.

The only downside of this scan was that it took three times longer than any of the previous ones. Elle took a real bruising and at one stage she was sent off to the loo to partially release the pressure on her swollen bladder. Ouch. The old spare part feeling returned with a vengeance as I watched, wincing with pain as the operator frantically thumped Elle's bump to try and get a better view.

Once we were done and packed off with yet more photos to add to our bumper collection, Elle began to feel pretty sick. I wasn't feeling too clever, either.

If I heave at the sight of Elle being gently poked by a nice lady just doing her job, how the hell am I going to cope with labour? Now that the 20 week mark has passed I can't help thinking that we're counting down to that fateful day.

If my overactive imagination is anything to go by, she'll be rushed in to the hospital ready to pop about 20 minutes after the first contraction. She'll squeeze my hand so tightly it will hurt, she'll call me a worthless bastard, scream and pant a bit, then she'll give birth to a flawless, clean and quiet baby at which stage I'll hand out cigars. Perhaps I can cope with that after all.

• • •

The midwife – our only friend in the harsh world of ante-natal care – had a really bad day today and left us both feeling crap.

First, she again failed to come up with the results of bloods Elle gave ages ago, second she failed to find a heartbeat, leading to more prodding, bruising and bashing for Elle. Finally she listened with a gaping mouth as Elle was forced to explain the new maternity rights and demand a form to claim her maternity pay before it is too late. The midwife wandered off to ask a colleague who was also bemused by the changes in mothers' rights, but in the end she gave in, gave us the form and sent us away. Thank God we didn't start on paternity rights.

Get what's coming to you
Paternity pay

Now is the time to find out what you're entitled to in the way of paternity leave. The money won't set your world alight but it has improved a bit since the Work and Families Act, which came into force in April 2007. And it does mean that you can get a bit of extra leave without breaking the bank. If you've been employed by a company for at least six months without a break up to the 15th week before the baby's due date, your minimum entitlement is two weeks leave on what is known as statutory pay. You only get the money if you earn more than a certain amount (£90 a week gross in 2008/9) and the maximum money you can get is capped to a maximum (£117.18, 2008/9)or 90 per cent of earnings if your pay is less than that figure. Also, employed fathers now have the right to take up to 26 weeks Additional Paternity Leave, some of which could be paid if your partner returns to work.

You have to tell your employer when you want the leave by the 15th week before the baby is due (probably when your partner is about 25 weeks pregnant) and the claim must be made using a self-certification form. You can download one of these forms, and get access to all the latest information on leave and entitlements, from the employee section of **www.direct.gov.uk**

It is so depressing to be buggered around by her because she's supposed to be the only person who's fighting from our corner. I'm not questioning her ability, or the skill of any of the medical staff we've come across. But I'd like a bit more understanding of the fact that it is all new to us – new and frightening. When something goes wrong, or a test is delayed or forgotten, I'd like to know why, not because I'm pushy, but because it matters.

It might be stupid to expect to be kept informed and updated at all times – that might be asking too much of a stretched NHS. But in reality all I'm asking is that people who deal with pregnancy day after day in their working lives respect the fact that we don't. For us this is unique and special, and there's no reason they can't accept that. It costs nothing and it means everything.

Chapter Seven
Your changing lives

"Whatever you think when you see her looking massive, tired and sweaty, remember that it's not her choice to be like this. Tell her that you love her and that she looks great." L, dad of three

---

What's happening?

Month seven

Your partner's symptoms – as the baby's weight increases your partner will be feeling the strain in two key areas. Firstly, she may be suffering from more pronounced back pain and discomfort in the ribs and sides – this can only really be eased by resting and good posture, though if the pain becomes more intense, your partner should talk to her midwife or doctor about arranging a physiotherapy appointment at the hospital. The second area where she'll feel the pinch is in her bladder, which is now being squeezed almost out of existence. That means many trips to the loo, so try to make sure you're never far away from one.

Your baby – brain function is now increasing as the central nervous system becomes more complex. Smart kid!

Elle is well over the halfway stage of pregnancy, she has a bump that would draw admiring nods at the World Darts Championships and the summer has come up with its first heatwave – all of which has added to her feeling of discomfort.

The bump hasn't seemed large until now, not because it hasn't been there, but simply because it isn't something I've thought much about. It has slowly appeared and now it is a part of life, making Elle walk a bit oddly, giving her a bit more difficulty when bending down and picking stuff up. But generally she wears it well. Some men don't like the shape of a pregnant woman, and I guess I can understand that, it's a part of the realisation that your partner is changing from the girl you know into a mother, maybe even into *her* mother. Put it that way and it scares the shit out of me, too.

Some men go the other way and find pregnancy a complete turn-on. Though I've never gone down this route, I'm told there are even porn magazines devoted solely to pregnant women. Yes, well.

Elle's gone away on a management course. She told me on the phone last night that one of their tasks was to set personal objectives for the next six months. She didn't know whether she should write 'have a baby'.

Life is pretty weird for her right now. She's good at her job in spite of all the men around her – mainly because she's always been able to be accepted as one of 'the blokes'. But pregnancy changes all that. Some of the men have adapted well, some haven't. They all seem to treat her slightly differently and that has bothered her. Many of her colleagues are dads, so they can look back on their own experiences. Little jokes about forgetfulness and hormones might seem pretty harmless, but I can see how much it upsets her to think they are questioning whether she can do her job properly. All of a sudden, she's unsure about who she is.

I feel the same. This short window of independence is most likely the last time we'll be apart before the baby is born. In the run up to these few days, I've had plenty of plans – to lounge around in my underwear, get drunk in the morning, watch a pile of crappy films, write a crappy play – spread out, be selfish, fart a lot and enjoy my last few days of hedonistic independent living.

It is now 8pm. Elle has rung me, I've eaten my dinner, washed up and now I'm settling down with a small glass of beer. So far today I've managed to do the washing, the ironing and the vacuuming. I've walked the dogs a few times, posted a letter and had a bath, making sure to clean it thoroughly afterwards. Woah, there. Wild man.

OK, so I'm now a stranger to wild living. Responsibility creeps up on you from the minute you agree to share a house with someone, for reasons that are both financial and emotional. If you get a pet, you're tied even more. We have four pets, not counting the birds in the garden and the mice in the walls. It turns out that I'm already a family man, whether I'm prepared for it or not.

Keeping it together

Your relationship and your identity

Everything might be baby, baby, baby around now, but it doesn't hurt to remind yourself why you got into this situation in the first place – and before you say 'because the condom split' I'm talking about love. Because you do, hopefully, love your partner and may well hope to spend the rest of your lives together. Contrast this long-lasting relationship with the fickle little soul who's about to interrupt the flow of your twosome only to disappear off to share a flat with some unsuitable mates in Stevenage in eighteen years' time. Put it this way, and suddenly it makes sense to be sure that you're in both emotional places at the same time. So how do you keep the love in your life? Here's how:

Be romantic. Remember what life was like when you were trying to impress her? Well, it won't do you any harm to hark back to that time now. Buy her flowers or a gift that makes her feel special. You could even just do something spontaneous like cooking her a candle-lit meal. Whatever you do, she'll appreciate the gesture and even if she reacts by bursting into tears or saying she couldn't eat a bite of the delicious meal you've slaved over simply smile and say you understand. She's not 100 per cent in control of her emotions and you both need to be aware of this and cut each other some slack.

Make time. Your relationship will soon be suffering from a serious squeeze in quality time, so you need to establish the rule of 'ring-fenced' couple time right now. In fact it's good practice to establish this dedicated time right up to the birth and carry it on immediately beyond. Even if you just have an hour out together for lunch you are both making a clear statement that you value each other and want to be together.

Have a break. Now's a good time to go away together – you may not get the chance for a while after the birth. If you're going abroad, your partner should be careful about food and especially drinks overseas, and you should ensure that your travel insurance covers pregnancy. Don't leave it too late to travel, most airlines won't accept bookings from women who are more than 32 weeks pregnant.

Respect each other. I know it sounds obvious, but you do both need to acknowledge that you're going through this together. If either of you feels excluded from anything in the pregnancy – whether it's you feeling like an outsider around tests, scans and midwife checks or her feeling sidelined by exhaustion – then there will be problems ahead. Talk together at every stage and help each other through it. If you work as a team, I guarantee you'll survive the experience intact.

Don't expect a sense of humour. No matter how charming and witty you are, you're going to get a clunk round the side of the head with a frying pan if you compare your partner in maternity gear to an elephant wearing a marquee. And you'll deserve it. The side-splitting jokes should be reserved for junior's first birthday.

Do it together. Again, this might sound obvious, but parents-to-be often get carried away by the sheer volume of things to be done – buying stuff, decorating, even moving house or changing jobs, and they end up dividing the work up and as a result they see almost nothing of each other in the process. Don't fall into this trap, do the baby stuff together wherever possible and try to make it more fun and less of a chore.

Don't be a chore bore. And finally, if you do end up doing everything for her because she can't manage it herself, don't make a big deal of it and/or expect too much gratitude – as with the comment on sense of humour failure above, you're not likely to get much sympathy if you start moaning about how tough your life has become.

• • •

I am so glad that Elle is back from her course. Not just because it means I can stop feeling so much pressure to do something wild in her absence, but because I worry about her every movement. I spend so much time imagining possible problems and traumas that it becomes a great relief to see her fit and well at the end of each day.

And she is well. Not only that, she's actually blooming. She's decided that she'll take a bit of holiday that's owing then start maternity leave early, basically giving up work at 30 weeks. It's a big relief for me, but a bigger one for her – she's been totally split between wanting to do a good job and wanting to get on with the whole baby thing.

She gets a pile of e-mails every day from pushy baby product manufacturers, trying to pass on vital knowledge and shift a few nappies into the bargain. Each of these has general tips for well-being and a few points on what to look out for. My favourite one arrived this morning. It said something along the lines of 'don't be disturbed if your partner starts to behave differently. He may take up a hobby, like woodwork, or grow a moustache'. Come on, you people, how many men have actually reacted to the news that they're going to be a dad by growing facial hair? And woodwork?

"Darling, I'm pregnant."

"That's wonderful darling. And look, I've made a pipe rack."

"You animal. Come here, I want to feel your stubble against my cheek."

I get the general message that is coming across here – men tend to act more grown-up in response to the coming demands of fatherhood. Most blokes I know feel they aren't ready for the new arrival, that they still have plenty of growing up to do themselves. That's quite right and totally human. But woodwork? Moustaches? God no, please don't let it be true.

I should add at this stage that my disbelief has nothing to do with the fact that I was kicked out of woodwork at school and have always been cursed with a thin beard. It's just grade A bullshit, pure and simple.

"And we call this a nappy..."
Dealing with stereotypes

It might be bullshit, but it is a part of a wider problem that you've probably already started to come up against, and will certainly have to deal with as the due date approaches. You are about to be stereotyped, bracketed, patronised and talked down to on a scale not seen since you had that maths teacher with BO in the third year. It'll come from everywhere – from parents who've done it all, from medical professionals, from books and from TV.

You are a buffoon, a complete idiot who forgets to pack the bag, gets lost in the hospital, puts on nappies back to front, passes out in the delivery suite etc, etc. Think of every cliché and comic image of dads-to-be, and you'll be stuck with almost all in the next couple of months. Is this a bad thing? It depends on your reaction. If it angers you, then it's bad. If you start to believe it, that's a tragedy. But low expectations could give you the space you need to get confident about your role before and after the birth. After all, if everyone's expecting you to fall flat on your face, every little success will feel great.

• • •

For the last few weeks Elle has been feeling serious movements from the baby. They started about six weeks ago as a kind of fluttering and have been building up ever since. While it was still new, she'd shout to me to come and feel her belly. By the time I got there, the baby was done stretching and had settled back to sleep, or it had shifted enough to start booting her spine instead.

But recently the kicks have been so powerful that I've been able to feel them too. It's such a weird feeling, and so hard to imagine the little foot or elbow that's stretching Elle's skin and fighting for a bit more room inside. In one way it's great to be able to feel and see the growth of the child, but in another it also shows the fact that I'm just an outsider to this strange double act.

Elle's even started to detect a pattern of waking and sleeping at fixed times. The baby's most awake at about 3am, but I'm hoping it'll grow out of it. I'm a bit jealous of the strong and natural closeness that's building up between my wife and child.

The other downside of a regular pattern of kicks and punches is that I get into an immediate panic if Elle says the baby has gone quiet. I really should have got hold of that portable ultrasound monitor – I bet I could have picked one up on e-Bay.

This happened just yesterday. Elle went off to work like normal, but through breakfast, she'd been worried about the fact that she hadn't felt the baby move for a few hours. I wanted her to stay at home, maybe go into the hospital for a scan, but we looked at the books again and they said it wasn't always something to worry about. After about 28 weeks, it's meant to be normal to pick up around 10 clear movements every day, but until then the odd lengthy period without a flinch isn't a big worry.

Unfortunately, the worst part of working from home is that you've got nothing to distract you from worrying that there is a real problem. With mum and child half an hour away at work, all I could do was sit and fret. Well, that was my excuse for playing computer games all day.

Is there anybody there?

Getting help and guidance

If you want to avoid being talked down to by smug new dads – who a few short months ago were crapping themselves in your shoes (as it were) – your options for expressing and voicing your fears are limited. While it's good to talk to your partner, you might want to check the facts a bit before you get her involved with something that turns out to be totally irrelevant. Your fears might also be about her, of course. Childless mates won't be a lot of use, so the only real hope comes from other fathers-to-be.

The question is, how do you get to speak to them? Some may go to antenatal classes (which we'll look at later in the book) but these are often held late on in the pregnancy. There are a few message boards online for dads only, but a glance through some of the more popular boards suggests that they are often invaded by mums-to-be, so they aren't generally too open and frank.

The truth – and the reason for this book's existence – is that true understanding is hard to find. I was lucky enough to have a couple of mates going through the process around the same time as me, but even then I didn't share experiences with them as often as I could, and should, have done. The fact is that you will get through by relying on a variety of different sources – an informative web site, a good book, some decent mates, an understanding partner. They can all help, but not one of them can give you all the answers.

Of course, Elle came home and reported that she'd gone 12 rounds with the little thug during a vital business meeting and I breathed a sigh of relief. I really, really should get out more.

•   •   •

Now I am getting out more. In a week Elle is going to pass over the baton to me as she starts her maternity leave and

I start tutoring at a summer school in a local college. It's only seven weeks, but it gives me the chance to get out from under the towering and scary heap of baby clothes catalogues that has appeared next to the sofa. I'm glad to be doing it. I love Elle, but our conversation rarely moves away from the baby. This is made worse by the fact that this phase of pregnancy is known by most of the blokes I know as the dull bit – the long stroll into the scary home straight.

Playing catch-up

Occupying yourself in the home straight

Do you remember that feeling from school of having holiday homework which you left untouched for weeks, only to find that you had to do it all in one terrifying Sunday afternoon? That's the same feeling you'll get if, like me, you regard this time as 'the dull bit'. With me at work and Elle stuck at home, hot and virtually unable to move, it was very hard to manage the large number of things we still hadn't done. We had to buy a car seat, a pram and a million other bits and bobs in a blind panic before time ran away from us completely. It might sound really dull, but now is also the time to get cracking on all those major DIY jobs that need doing after the baby's born. For the first three months of the kid's life you'll have no time to even consider such things, so get them in now while the world is moving at a gentle pace.

It'll also be good to get back into traditional roles for a while, especially if we decide to stay in them after the baby's born. I sometimes wonder whether after a couple of years of working from home I've become a weird hermit-like freak of nature who can't speak to his fellow men. At least I'll be at home in the world of education.

Chapter Eight
Getting ready for the birth

"Towards the end of pregnancy, women become very dependent, and maternity leave is often started after the birth but should be considered way before."
G, dad of two

What's happening?
Month eight.

Your partner's symptoms – your partner's changing shape can affect her in strange ways. As she's now accommodating a sizeable lump inside her, she may be walking or standing differently to normal which can have a knock-on effect on her joints, but it can also affect her balance. If she feels faint or woozy at this late stage it's because her centre of gravity is completely thrown by the imminent arrival. She won't be able to bend and stretch so well, so you might have to help with simple tasks like putting on shoes and socks.

Your baby – movements from the baby will be less pronounced because the poor little blighter is running out of room. Your partner should still feel regular movements, but they will be more in the form of shifts and wriggles rather than sharp jabs and upper cuts to the ribcage.

When I was a kid, every summer I was treated to a trip to Dreamland amusement park in Margate. There was nothing particularly dreamlike about the place, though it felt like it had been asleep for about 100 years. The rides weren't exactly white-knuckle, more white-haired.

My favourite was the Scenic Railway, a sort of flat roller coaster that ran round the outside of the park. It was slow and steady, but sometimes the cart would jump on the warped and buckled tracks and there was an occasional slight hill that took an age to climb up to as the carts were ratcheted up a notch only to slide feebly down the other side.

I've thought about that ride all through this pregnancy.

There's no doubt I've felt that I'm on some kind of con-
veyor belt, that there's no going back or straying from the
path. It's also true there's been the odd lump and bump
along the way. Generally, though, it's been steady all the
way. But now, hitting 30 weeks is like starting the slow
and boring climb before the shit scary drop into the
unknown territory of labour and birth. How do I take this
plunge without losing my lunch?

Smart arses may argue that it is the woman who faces the
bigger deal at this stage, but I say bullshit to that. My role
is to stand on the sidelines and not interfere, not panic
and not fall backwards over expensive monitoring equipment. It's not easy, and I need to be shown how to keep
myself calm, cool and upright.

Ante-natal classes start next week, and I've got a free afternoon, so I'm going to go along to the first session. In my
head I have a picture of a room full of women sitting on
floor cushions breathing deeply and trying not to piss
themselves, but I'm sure the reality is less appealing.

I need these classes badly. Over the last couple of weeks
Elle has been wising up on pregnancy in general, thanks
to the Pregnancy Channel or some such cable crap. She's

also read every book available while pinned to the sofa by heat and tiredness. She keeps asking me questions about different pain relief methods and birth positions. I hadn't expected to be involved in this part of the decision making process, after all she's the one going through the pain, so I've guessed it's been up to her. If she wants drugs, give her drugs, I say. I'd want drugs. So far I've bluffed my way through it but I badly need a different answer from "which do you think is best?" quickly followed by, "yes, that's what I was going to go for".

A lack of understanding of the subject can be dangerous in other ways. This reminds me of the story about the American woman who heard a medical term during labour that she thought was so beautiful, she picked it as a name for her daughter. You've no chance in life when you are called Meconium[1].

I don't want to put in the hours of research and bad TV Elle has gone through, but if I'm going to be take part in decision making I don't want to appear as thick as pig shit. What I need is clear, non-patronising, simple and effective

---

[1] *It means newborn baby shit – I looked it up.*

advice on the reality of the delivery suite. And where better to find it than at NHS antenatal classes?

•   •   •

I am never, ever going to another antenatal class in my life. OK, so that's mainly because I don't have any more free afternoons, but I'd also have to say that the experience was a complete nightmare.

For starters it was just about the hottest day of the year so far, and the class was held in one of those rooms built in the 1970s as a large scale model of a microwave oven. We sat and dripped sweat everywhere as the presiding health care woman – I never actually heard her job title – told us that there wouldn't be a midwife present due to ill health.

This woman was there to talk to us about breathing techniques, pain relief and other key subjects. I mentally rubbed my hands – actually rubbing them together would have led to a sticky, sweaty mess – this was exactly the stuff I'd wanted to hear.

Unfortunately, I was the only partner who did want to hear it. As the only representative in the room of a species that all the other hot, angry participants were slowly beginning to resent, I felt pretty awkward.

Fortunately, the tension was ended by our hostess who singled me out while cracking such classic gags as "when the second stage of labour begins, you should really try not to be watching the football on TV, dad".

"I'll try," I said feebly as the women around me snorted with utter contempt. "Just as surely as I'll try not to fling my chair across the room at your fat, ugly head," I added, in the car on the way home.

In between those comments I sat quietly and nodded along as required. I did the breathing exercise and I tried to soak up as much detail as I could. It was useful and informative, but I got the feeling that I wasn't entirely welcome. That's odd, and what's even odder is the decision of our health authority to cancel the final, evening session of the antenatal classes which many working fathers could have attended. Again I'm met with the feeling that the medical staff feel men are going to be no real use, so should be sidelined at all costs.

I'm pretty sure that's not a view shared by most mothers-to-be, so the only reason for it must just be that it is tradition. But as our midwife said, in the course of her 30-something years in the job, the tradition has gone from seeing fathers in the delivery room as freaks to the complete opposite. Traditions change, that's the great thing about evolution, that and the fact we no longer live in trees and eat bugs. So somewhere down the line, the man is going to have to be seen by the system as a key partner in pregnancy.

A class apart

Getting the best out of antenatal classes

I'm pleased to say that there are many health authorities a good deal smarter than ours, and these hold classes in the evenings or at times suitable to working fathers. If your health authority doesn't, it's probably because of a mixture of staffing issues and a deep held belief that fathers-to-be wouldn't be fussed about going.

But good antenatal classes are a great preparation for your role in the delivery suite, and you shouldn't let the opportunity go by without a fight. So if you can't get time off, complain, and get others to do the same. If they won't change the time, then the very least they should do is hold one dedicated session that deals with issues for men. If you do get to attend a session, you should expect to learn more about the following:

The signs and stages of labour. The class leader (usually a midwife or a nurse or health visitor) will talk you through the signs and symptoms of the onset of labour as well as the procedure for getting booked into the delivery suite (if you are having a hospital delivery). She will also explain the stages of labour and explain any other terminology or issues that may arise (see chapter 9 for a more detailed explanation).

Pain relief in labour. While your partner may only decide on the type of pain relief to choose once the contractions kick in, there's a good opportunity here to find out more about the merits of the various options. This can be particularly useful if your partner is going to create a birth plan, a written record of her plans, hopes and expectations for the birth which should be passed to the midwives on arrival at the delivery suite (again, there's more information on pain relief options in chapter 9).

Breathing and relaxation techniques. For women who choose to avoid or limit pain relieving drugs, the natural alternative is to use breathing control techniques. The class leader will show your partner how to breathe in through her nose and out through her mouth during contractions. If you follow the instruction, you stand a better chance of being able to guide your partner through when it counts on the big day.

Another vital relaxation technique that you can learn at antenatal classes is how to use massage to help ease the lower back pain of your partner when contractions get really intense.

Babies. Ok, so this might be jumping the gun a little bit, but when you think about it, the antenatal class is the last occasion you are going to get to learn about childcare before you're actually thrown into the bearpit itself. So if the class leader is prepared to give some instruction on basics like feeding, changing and bathing a baby, you'll earn brownie points by listening now.

Go private. If you really like the idea of getting access to a decent support network prior to the birth, you might want to complement the slightly impersonal but free NHS antenatal classes with some private classes, either those run by the NCT, or by a local parents' group. The downside is that you have to pay for the privilege of sitting on a pouffe and panting like a dog, but the upside is that you get into the delivery suite brim full of confidence.

• • •

The antenatal class helped me feel a little less woozy, but it hasn't lasted. A couple of days down the line and Elle has come back from another midwife check-up with a new and totally unexpected change of plan. She wants to have the baby at home.

Oh shit. As soon as she mentioned it, I realised two things – she is dead set on the idea, and I hate the idea more than anything in the world. This is a major problem.

My fears are simple and, I think, justified. Our house, lovely and comfortable though it is, has no medical facilities. The midwives who have seen Elle to date in pregnancy are either unpredictable or extremely inexperienced. To trust the delivery of our baby to these kindly yet bumbling folks would be utterly stupid. I can picture a huge range of nightmare scenarios in which we are faced with medical emergencies beyond our wildest fears and all I can do is boil water and serve up platefuls of biscuits as we wait for nature to sort out the mess. No, no and no. Over my dead body. End of story.

•   •   •

Not quite. Now that I come to think of it, a home birth might be quite a good idea, after all. OK, so I've still got a few minor doubts, but after think it over it's growing on me. Why the change of heart? I've spoken to a few parents in the last couple of days, and the responses have been amazingly similar. All the men have shaken their heads accompanied by that 'tut-tut-tut' beloved of mechanics. All the women have said that they wished they'd had home births. A large number actually did. They survived, their kids survived and maybe, just maybe it wasn't all by accident. Sixty years ago it was your only option, after all.

So I realized that it is only men who have a real problem with home births. But why? Take our situation, we're just a few miles from the hospital, so if anything was to go wrong, we'd be seen as soon as possible. The positive effect of the relaxed home environment could be a real bonus in a long labour. I'd have all my home comforts and I could even make meals and drinks. But the nagging doubts don't just go away, no matter how good the evidence appears. I claim that it's because I want to be sure that Elle and the baby are getting the best care throughout the process, but these fears are mine, they are about me and the level of guilt and responsibility I'd feel if something went wrong because I hadn't put my foot down. When do I accept that I should let go and just give Elle the support she needs to make the right decision for herself?

Later. I can take the chicken shit option of waiting, because if she goes into labour early, she goes into hospital, no question. If she goes past 37 weeks, we can have the debate then. Yeah, that'll work. You arsehole.

•   •   •

Without either of us actually saying so, we've agreed that our sex life has come to an end until after the birth. We both have our reasons – Elle is suffering a lot with discomfort in her hips and pelvis as the baby grows and I'm more than a little spooked by the idea of being kicked by the baby in the heat of passion. I've always been a bit shy in the sexual arena, but bring in an audience and I'm totally shafted, so to speak.

Of course, if it wasn't for Elle's physical pain and my shyness, we could be happily shagging away until the baby is due. It doesn't harm the baby and it does a lot to ease the stress of the final few weeks.

Left hand down a bit

Sex in pregnancy (part two)

Sex at this stage in pregnancy is an art form, like a very sweaty game of Twister. It is all about positions and communication – even though you won't hurt the baby, you'll probably end up hurting yourself or your partner if things aren't well planned in advance. Here's a guide to getting the best out of sex in the final weeks.

Position is king. We aren't talking about running all the way through the Kama Sutra here, just a slight move away from the old-fashioned missionary position. Trust me when I say that getting her to lie flat on her back for hours while you steam away above her is not sexy. It might just about qualify as preparation for the long and boring period in the delivery room, but that wouldn't do you any favours as a lover. You are still pretty safe with her on top, because she can keep control – though having your belly slapped by a huge bulge is a bit too much like Sumo for most men. Your best bet is either the side-on 'spoons' position (good sensation, fairly shallow penetration) or all fours (which achieves very deep penetration which can be very stimulating late in pregnancy but which can also get quite tiring for her).

Breast aware. Again, it's worth noting that those tits, which by now will be on the way to being full of milk, are going to be fairly sensitive. So handle with care.

Bring it on. Sex in late pregnancy is one of the more believable old wives' remedies for bringing on an overdue labour. While the act of intercourse isn't going to actually start labour, there is some scientific evidence behind this idea. A hormone in your sperm can help to soften the cervix (mouth of the uterus) while stimulation of the nipples and clitoris can help push your partner closer to labour, especially if she climaxes. Hell, you might as well give it a try.

When we stopped having sex for a while earlier in the pregnancy, it was all my fault. I didn't know what to do or say for the best. I was worried that I'd harm the baby, or that I'd hurt Elle. If I'd talked to her more openly it might have eased things. But this time, though we don't really speak openly about the subject, there's been lots of communication. She is suffering – tired, sore and a bit irritable. She lets me know, with gentle nudges and firm kicks, that I should be getting back into hired slave mode. Not being around all the time makes that hard, but when I am home, I try to be helpful.

A lot of what she's going through is beyond my help. The

worst thing is the tiredness, I'd guess. Not only does she find lying down uncomfortable, she has to get up all the time in the night to pee. Sometimes I wonder if nature is just a great big hidden camera stunt, designed to make people look really dumb. It certainly seems awfully cruel at times.

"Are you awake?"

Her changing sleep pattern

A couple of months later, when the experience had the rosy glow of hindsight, Elle described a typical night to me. She'd get into bed, shift herself onto her side, tuck a pillow between her legs and drop off straight away. An hour or so later she'd wake, stiff as a board and desperate to change position. She'd have to sit up, remove the pillow, move herself painfully onto her other side, then set it all up again, only to discover that she needed to have a piss.

It was a miracle that I stayed asleep with all that going on next to me. It's a hard time for your partner, her womb is doing its best to flatten her bladder, so it fills in no time, and this, the aches and pain, kicks and movements are keeping her awake. What can you do about it? Not a lot – if she's at home and filling her day with chores you could take on a few more, freeing her up for a guilt-free afternoon nap. You could buy her a shaped pillow (you can get these from specialist baby and mother care shops) that supports her body.

Your main task is to remove all the little stresses – bills, families, shopping, cleaning, washing – that she can't deal with while she's putting up with all the crap nature is hitting her with. Relaxation and breathing techniques work for some women, and as she's well past the six months stage of pregnancy, you could get her some aromatherapy oils or salts for a chill out late night bath. Check with the shop that the ones you're getting are suitable for pregnancy.

We keep getting messages from friends and family saying that we should be getting all the sleep we can at this stage 'because we're really going to need it after'. Thanks, guys. Big help.

Dream on

Your changing sleep pattern

Actually, it is good advice. I wish I'd taken it. If she can't sleep, you won't help her by staying awake in sympathy. As one of the surveyed fathers explained, sleep is going to be at a premium from onset of labour until God knows when. You need yours now.

•　•　•

Now that the summer school has finished, I'm back home full time. It's just as well, Elle's mobility has been getting a lot worse over the last few weeks, and now she can't drive or walk the dogs. I am needed more than ever and I think that is probably a bit annoying for her. For me, it's a taste of what's to come, a hint of the future.

I've been thinking a lot about becoming a dad. It still feels like quite an alien idea, but I find myself wondering again what sort of a father I'll be. My own dad has always been caring without being too emotional. He's always stepped back when I want to be free and stepped forwards when I want help. I could do a lot worse.

And yet I want to be a bit different. For starters I want to be more hands-on than my dad was. I want to take on care a bit more equally, though of course I haven't the faintest idea about the reality of looking after a baby. I might hate the idea when it comes to it. But I want to try. If I screw up then I can try my hand at something else, like gardening or collecting vintage toy cars.

Maybe I just shouldn't think about it at all. If, as everyone never tires of telling me, I am going to be taken completely by surprise, then I should just sit back and let it happen. A good friend of mine set about fatherhood with all the mistaken good intentions of a DIY enthusiast trying to build a Swedish wardrobe. He found himself totally confused by the resulting balls-up. There are no instructions, no map, no easy answers, just experience and trial and error.

·   ·   ·

It looks like my cowardly plan to put off the home birth debate has worked, though to be honest, I wish it hadn't. The reason a home birth is ruled out is that Elle's painful hip is worse than ever. She's been given crutches by the hospital physiotherapist and is really struggling to get around. It's a really miserable situation, made all the more crap by the fact that we can't go anywhere or do anything that takes her mind off her discomfort.

We're in some kind of bizarre Groundhog Day situation at the hospital, we keep going to see the consultant, who is never there, and his registrars keep telling us that everything's fine and Elle should be OK for a natural birth. The only trouble is that while they all agree on this point, one of them thinks an epidural painkiller would be a good idea, while another thinks it would cause more damage. The physiotherapist doesn't want to get involved and the others don't want to commit. And absolutely no one seems to have any suggestions for dealing with the pain now.

I hate the hospital. I didn't like the sight of it on that first terrible visit ages ago for the emergency scan and I still despise it. What I hate most of all is the fact that my wife is forced to sit for hours on end, only to repeat her story to every new face she sees. By now, there are tears of frustration in her eyes each time we visit and nothing is done. All we see is a stream of people who have good explanations for why it isn't their fault or their responsibility. When we started seeing the consultants, I felt a bit odd watching them wrestle with Elle's belly and abdomen, especially the men. As a partner you're not normally part of these essential but very personal dealing with someone else. I wouldn't say I've been feeling jealous, but I have started to get more protective, especially as the examinations have become more painful.

As Elle has got more stressed and frustrated by the endless

line of doctors, I've been able to use a successful tactic from my dealings with the midwife. We talk about everything before each appointment and I generally make a list of all the questions we want answered. Elle is rarely in the right state of mind to remember everything, so I provide a pretty good back-up.

Even the moody hospital receptionists are starting to recognise Elle by her distinctive limp and pained expression. We've started to get something close to human sympathy from them. Secretly I think this has less to do with Elle's plight and more to do with the fact that admin people always love to get one over on their professional colleagues. They tut sadly as we explain how hard it is to get anyone to take us seriously, then promise to do all they can to fight on our behalf – perhaps by ordering the wrong sort of paper clips or something.

One thing they have done is to make sure that we can been seen by the actual consultant at our next appointment. Though whether he'll make any difference remains to be seen.

• • •

He's made a difference. He listened and seemed to know how to respond, how to put our minds at ease, but more than anything else he made a difference by deciding that Elle's wait has been long and painful enough. He booked her in for induction of labour next week. Next week? Oh shit.

She'll be at full term according to our dates, but it's still one hell of a shock to the system to know that she's now a ticking time bomb. The moment she goes into the delivery suite, she is staying there until the baby is born. In other words, I'm going to be a father in a matter of days.

Cue panic. I am the least prepared dad-to-be in the whole world. There must be a bag to pack. No, there's two bags to pack, one for Elle, one for the baby. But what to put in? So far my mental list consists of the following – toy for the baby, hat for the baby bought from football club shop (size six months plus), copy of the Radio Times and chocolate bars. To my surprise none of these items are on the official list which Elle patiently gave me. Except for the hat, but not this hat, I could use this hat as a carry cot.

Calm down. Everything is under control, magically purchased by the shopping fairies. We've got little bodysuits and sleep suits and non-gender specific clothes and socks, boots, mittens, sheets, towels. The baby's bag is bigger than Elle's – a taste of what's to come, I fear. Elle's bag is filled with clothes that look like something from a Victorian Ann Summers party, heavy black dresses with holes in the chest where she can stick the baby's head without causing distress in public by forcing men to stare at her breasts. These weird clothes are about as interesting as the pre-birth maternity gear she's had to wear, most of which is shapeless and dark, none of which is any good in the summer. At least she's never had to wear dungarees.

We've given the dogs to Elle's parents, who are, understandably, nervous and excited about the big event. We made this decision to give them something to do because it takes their minds off things, but it also keeps them tied safely to their home 100 miles away. After weeks of softening them up for the news, we've finally explained that we won't be expecting to see them at the hospital – in fact all relatives, friends and well-wishers are banned until we get home again. On the plus side that means I get quality time with Elle and the baby, on the minus side it means I'm on my own if things go wrong.

I don't want to think about that. I've packed the bags, checked and rechecked everything and even placed them hopefully at the bottom of the stairs. Now all I have to do is wait for a week until Elle goes in to hospital.

"So where's the pool table?"
Visiting the delivery suite

If your partner's going to have a hospital delivery, there's a good chance that the maternity wing will let the pair of you have a wander round the place to get familiar with the layout. These tours are normally held once a week in groups. They'll almost certainly be on a weekday, which means more time off work, but it's worth it. You'll be feeling pretty lost when you're there for real, so this dry run just gives you an idea of where the bogs are and whether there's a place to make a coffee or a snack.

Waiting with a goal in sight is easily better than life before the consultant. Until the decision to induce, Elle faced another month of misery. All she has to cope with now is a few days of watching me race around like an idiot.

Pull yourself together man

Getting organised

While I was faffing around with my headless chicken act, there was a load of useful things I could have been doing. It would have been good to get hold of a plan of the hospital – parking was always a nightmare, and I didn't have a clue where to take her in an emergency. Similarly, I hadn't made any emergency travel plans in case the direct route to the hospital was blocked. I didn't have the midwife's emergency number in my wallet, nor did I have the numbers of friends and family. They're all simple things, but they need attention, and it'll make both you and your partner feel at ease if you've got them covered.

This is also the time to catch up on any essential shopping, including getting enough food for you and your partner for a week or so after she comes out of hospital.

Of course, she'd really like it to be over now, and I have to balance my desire to put it off until I'm a grown-up with the wish to see the baby and end Elle's suffering. The midwife at the hospital said we should try a few old tricks to bring the baby on. Her first two suggestions were long walks and lots of sex, which almost got her a clump round the head with a crutch, but then she quickly added the other ideas of hot curries and raspberry leaf tea. Not one of these remedies are actually official medical opinion, but they do make good common sense. Walking and sex keep you healthy and lithe, a hot curry is a shock to the system and raspberry tea is so horrible you want to give birth just to avoid drinking another drop. But then, as Elle pointed out after my third cup, she's the one who is supposed to drink the tea.

In all honesty I'm hoping that none of these remedies work. I can deal with taking Elle into the hospital on a nice pre-planned, leisurely afternoon drive. But I don't fancy the thought of a bleary eyed midnight scramble, or a desperate call dragging me back from a meeting. We've had to turn down party invitations because they are too far from the hospital, and I've even cut back on the booze in the evenings, just in case I'm expected to drop everything at a moment's notice.

•   •   •

Another side-effect of spotting life at the end of the tunnel is that we've started to think about the baby again. For a couple of months Elle's well-being has dominated our thoughts. The baby has taken care of itself, as we have been assured it would.

But all that time, except for a few lost thoughts, we hadn't really thought about the person inside my wife's belly, the little stranger taking her strength, who is finally going to make an appearance.

Most of the talk had been about sex, which hasn't really been a hot topic since the anatomy scan. I'm still undecided, and I'd be happy to trust Elle's instinct on the subject, except she still doesn't seem to have one. In my heart I know that I'd cope better with a boy than a girl. I'm going to be overprotective in either case, but a boy might just stand half a chance of being independent. But having been a little boy myself, I can't help thinking what foul beasts they can be. Perhaps a girl would be better.

We're not really doing any better with names, though we've tried all sorts of scientific methods. We made a bit of a start months ago with a baby names book, scanning through page after page of names, calling out favourites. This quickly slipped into calling out the stupidest names we could find and pretty soon we gave up altogether. Now, though, I've got the book out again with serious intent and I've come up with a system where we go through it, writing down our top five in secret, then comparing answers to find the best placed option. Simple. Except our top fives featured totally different names. So it's back to square one. Some families pass on names like heirlooms, we don't have that simplicity of choice as I can't think of anyone in either of our immediate families who would actually want us to recycle their name. No, it's got to be our choice.

In this, as in most things, Elle has been the one who's had the more philosophical attitude. She says there's no point in finding and agreeing a name that might not fit the baby. So we'll hang on until we're properly introduced.

•   •   •

There's a couple of major, pressing issues that I just can't bring myself to discuss with Elle. The first, and worse, is something that has come from the endless cable show births that are ever present on our TV. It's something that keeps me awake all night. I absolutely, definitely don't want to cut the umbilical cord. This is a new tradition, and I'm sure a whole load of fathers have managed it and felt that it made them a real part of the delivery. But I really don't want to do it. It isn't out of fear, but out of pro-tection – I can't cut my own fingernails without slicing open an artery. If I'm pushed into doing anything med-ical, it'll be fatal for all concerned.

To be fair, I don't think it will take much to convince Elle of the logic of this decision. She's seen my attempts at DIY.

The other big fear is change. I'm not talking about my future here, just my coins. With a week to go before the big day, and with those bags packed, my only remaining useful function is to build up enough coins to pay for the hospital parking. I've turned into Rain Man. I keep count-ing the coins and putting them away, getting them out again, counting them again. It's hypnotic. And it helps to distract me from the fact that I am shit scared and under-prepared.

●   ●   ●

As if Elle hasn't had enough misery, her induction has now been delayed three times. We've been sat at home, packed and ready to go for days now. We don't really talk, there's an atmosphere of stress and frustration. All we do is sit, tense and alert, watching trash on TV and trying not to get each other worked up. It is the most horrible wait, though I have my precious coins for company. The hospital keep insisting that we call in every few hours to see if there's a spare bed. It is agony.

· · ·

The miracle finally happens. There's a bed. We're going in.

Chapter Nine
The big day arrives

"For me labour was hard – I wasn't asked about my feelings at all. It was traumatic as I was uncomfortable, felt sick, out of my depth and out of control. And I didn't eat for twelve hours." B, dad of one

"You need to be mentally prepared for your partner's labour – do something like smash your kneecap and then lock yourself in a room with her for 12 hours." L, dad of three

---

What's happening?

Month nine.

Your partner's symptoms – The baby's rapid growth means that your partner is likely to either be eating all the time just to keep her energy levels up or she's sleeping all the time to achieve the same result. She may be slowing down in preparation for the big day, or alternatively might be racing round with a paintbrush and a manic expression on her face. Either way, just let her get on with it.

Your baby – Over the course of the final month, your baby has put on weight at a frantic rate (sometimes up to 1oz per day) and is curled into a tight ball as the space in the uterus becomes increasingly cramped.

In total contrast to conception, labour is a slow process. We've spent the best part of five hours this evening sitting around in the God forsaken delivery suite, with Elle fixed up to a machine that measures exactly how far she is from the end of what is slowly becoming a living hell.

This endless wait is a total pain in the arse, especially as it's come hard on the heels of the equally long, equally frustrating wait to be allowed into the damned place to start with. I've read every single celebrity magazine written in the last six months and am now an expert on Jade's bowel movements (loose, frequent) and Jordan's implants (frequently loose). Elle is knackered, depressed and in pain. I'm just hungry and hot.

Why are hospitals so overheated? All the books tell us that a baby shouldn't be too hot, and God knows the poor pregnant women don't need any more warming up. Perhaps it is some kind of secret desire to make dads-to-be sweat, just so they'll think twice about ever shagging again, so they don't come back and use up more National Health resources. I've never been so uncomfortable and I'm not the one being poked and prodded by an assortment of midwives.

"Now, where did I put my trouser press?"
Your hospital survival kit

Like Elle, your partner will almost certainly get a long list of items to bring to hospital. These rarely include any seriously practical items for the men. Depending on your situation, you might be in the delivery suite or on the ward for a couple of days. Most men will be stuck in the place for a good 12 hour stretch before, during and after delivery. So you'll need to be properly organised:

Food and drink. Hospital facilities are generally pretty grim (think school meals without the nutritional value) and the shops and cafes generally open during regular hours only. Bring two or three chilled bottles of water, some energy snacks and plenty of fruit. Don't rely on crisps and sweets from the vending machine to get you through as these will give you a short-term sugar rush and a long-term headache.

Clothes. You'll need to dress like a mountaineer with plenty of layers – the heat of wards and delivery suites can be overwhelming, but you'll probably be glad of the chance to get some fresh air at some stage, especially if it's an all-nighter. Don't take too many valuables in with you as you may have to leave them in a locker room if you need to change into surgical gear (if your partner has a caesarean, for example).

Reading material. Even if your partner is already labouring, there may well be an incredible amount of sitting around involved, so stock up on books and magazines. Don't assume there will be any reading material at the hospital, and don't assume the shop will be open when you get there.

Gadgets. You'll need to remember a camera, which won't be high on your partner's priority list. Take a CD player or mp3 player – although it is nice to believe that you'll spend all your time whispering encouragement to your partner, that can become dull after the first day or so, and it can be a real lifesaver to drift off into some music to drown out the less appealing sounds of the delivery suite. Take a mobile phone in with you by all means, but don't expect to use it anywhere but outside. Even if it's pissing down, your loved ones probably won't settle for a quick text message. So you'll also need to take some change for the payphones.

One thing I've noticed in these long hours of being bored shitless is that hospital midwives are either huge or tiny. There seems to be no middle ground – perhaps they all start off large and sweat themselves down to withered, frail tiny elves. I certainly hope so.

The strangest part of this waiting game is knowing that it will end suddenly and dramatically. I'm worried about the pain Elle faces and I'm worried about the effort I'm going to have to put in to help her cope. I can suddenly see the great advantage in nipping off to the pub for a few hours and then coming back once the job's done. The idea of lots of alcohol is tempting right now, but not as tempting as the idea of avoiding all my responsibility and letting someone else deal with the whole mess.

Up on the ward, I'm worried about something other than the long wait or the high temperatures. Elle is, like most people, fairly private – especially at a time like this when she doesn't exactly feel like socialising. There's no alternative on this ward, however, a huge corridor of women moaning, groaning, snoring, crying and generally keeping each other awake. Elle's new temporary home is on an end section with one new mum and another mum-to-be. It's a horrid place, and, of course, it's hot as hell. As soon as she's settled I make my excuses and leave.

·　·　·

Back at home things are even worse. With the dogs at Elle's parents it's just me and the self-obsessed cats. One of them complained at me as I came into the dark, cold house. I just avoided stepping on a mouse she'd caught in the kitchen, while I scrambled around looking for some food. I settled on some crisps, chocolate, cold cuts and red wine. It's important to keep my strength up.

I have the place to myself. While this may normally be an opportunity to watch sport in the nude or try to make out the breasts on the scrambled adult channels while drinking beer from the bottle, I feel shattered. Instead of the above I had a long, hot bath and lay staring lazily at my sad, shrunken genitals. They are to blame, and they know it. I woke up with a start and sent a great splat of water over the bathroom floor, soaking the cat and making her run around with a surprising turn of speed.

Tomorrow is, more likely than not, the day on which my wife will give birth to our first child. The thought is so overwhelming that I just can't allow myself to think about it. Every time I let my mind wander over what lies ahead, I come back to the endless births we have watched on those shitty cable shows. Half of them are brutal natural deliveries in rough British inner cities, with knuckle-duster-wearing mothers swearing and sweating while their hideous, toothless husbands suck nervously on a roll-up in the waiting area. The other half are beautiful, overpopulated American delivery suite births where the baby slips out effortlessly and everyone hugs while the Pregnancy Planner gushes the words "good job" at the rosy cheeked, calm mother.

Somehow, I didn't imaging either scenario. In fact, I simply don't know what to expect at all. Whatever happened to being cool and prepared? This is like one of those dreams where you turn over the exam paper only to find the questions are all in Japanese. But I really can't afford to fail the test tomorrow.

Playing your part

How to handle the labour

Our surveyed fathers – most of whom went through natural deliveries with their partners – ranged in their experiences from feeling like a spare part who just got in the way, to a key part of the process. Generally it seems that the more prepared, relaxed and focused on your partner's needs you are, the better the experience. So what is likely to happen, and what can go wrong?

First signs. Most people think that labour begins with a 'show' – the plug of mucus which blocks the mouth of the uterus – or with breaking waters – the amniotic fluid from around the baby – or with contractions. In the first two cases, these signs don't automatically indicate the imminent onset of labour (though if her waters break early, seek medical advice). But if contractions start to come harder and faster, there's a strong chance that junior is on the way pretty soon.

In the delivery suite. Once contractions are very regular and strong (around every five minutes), your partner will need to go into the delivery suite (if she's having a hospital birth). The contractions are helping to widen the cervix – the mouth of the uterus. This process is known as the first stage of labour. Once the cervix is at least 10cm wide, your partner may be encouraged to push. When you're in the hospital, you partner may be offered pain relief, including gas and air (Entonox), the pain killer Pethedine or an epidural pain killing injection in the spine.

Second stage of labour. The second stage of labour is when your partner will have to put in all the hard work trying to push the baby out. This may be the stage where she is most in need of your encourage-ment and support, but don't be too phased if she seems to drift off into her own world. She will find her own way to cope with the pain and you'll simply need to be there to help out as necessary.

Assisted delivery. In an ideal world, the second stage of labour should lead neatly to the arrival of a healthy, screaming purple human, but sometimes nature needs a hand. Assisted deliveries give a mother a helping hand, either by use of metal forceps, which grip the baby's head from the sides so a doctor can pull while your partner pushes or a machine called a ventouse, which is like a small suction cap applied to the top of your baby's head. Neither method will harm the baby, but may cause a little damage to your partner's vagina.

Third stage of labour. Once the baby is delivered, the placenta needs to follow. This can be delivered naturally, but most women prefer to have the delivery of the placenta speeded up by an injection . Once this has happened the pain is over and you can all relax just a little.

• • •

Slept about four hours last night. Feel like shit. Feel much better than Elle, who had the typical night of unnecessary disturbance that only a hospital can offer.

She was sitting up, picking over some breakfast when I arrived. After about an hour of riveting conversation on the subject of my every waking movement away from her, I ran out of things to say. Sure, we could talk about the need to redecorate the bedroom, or the England football team's defensive problems, but this would be redundant small talk. The big issue is the baby, but neither of us feels like talking about it. The fact is that we've probably got 13 hours together to sit and dwell on where the hell this kid has got to.

A few hours later and there's not a lot to report. Elle has been for another examination and a further dose of the induction gel that's supposed to get things cracking. I've invented excuses to wander the halls of the hospital, wandering around the echoing corridors while gazing with barely concealed horror at the sheer range of things that can go wrong with the human body. A door smashed open with a terrible noise as a trolley appeared with its obligatory grey faced zombie – pushing another patient to theatre no doubt.

Scarier still was the scene that I witnessed in the main concourse of the hospital. The place has been decked out in fancy decorations and strewn with ghastly teddy bears in anticipation of the arrival of a couple of reality TV 'stars' who are coming to perform some celebrity CPR on the hospital's bank balance.

I must admit I was warned about this horror. Earlier this morning, the girl in the bed opposite Elle was babbling about some kind of cake sale the midwives were organising, as if they had time to spare from drinking coffee and smoking in the store cupboard. This girl is a reliable source, she appears to be a 'lifer', able to give a short statement on each member of the nursing staff – 'she's alright', 'watch her, she's a right bitch' etc. – as well as full biographical and biological details of the other inmates… sorry, patients. I get the feeling that if I bring her some smokes she might even be able to get Elle's labour speeded up. It may yet come to that.

So while I was stood in the foyer, watching hundreds of medical professionals distract themselves from their life saving jobs, I started to get even more nervous about what's to come. What if the person who's supposed to care for my wife and child is too busy fawning over some talentless prick out here?

As I'm unable to wrap my wife in cotton wool, I chose the next best thing and bought her a big bag of it from the pharmacy, and then got a pile of magazines and papers from the shop. When all else fails, read – it might take our minds off the prospect that our baby could well be delivered live on telly by some singing soap star.

"Fine, I'll just have to deliver it myself"
Remaining patient and positive

I can't guess your experience of labour, and I wouldn't try – but one thing I'm pretty sure you will experience is that huge feeling of powerlessness that was starting to overwhelm me as I waited around for something to happen. Whether it comes in the delivery suite itself or earlier there is a good chance that you'll find yourself anxious to get things moving, but unable to do a thing about it.

You need to accept that this is not what you are about at this stage – responsibility for that part of your partner's welfare has passed over to the hospital staff. But you can keep some control by ensuring that your partner's wishes for the birth are met. If she's made a birth plan – a list of practical dos and don'ts like whether to have pain killing drugs in labour or a jab to help deliver the placenta – make certain you have a copy and that you know what it all means.

We wrote a plan that detailed Elle's pelvic and hip problems, made multiple copies of it and stuffed it into every face we saw. The woman who ran the antenatal class described how women rise to a higher plane in the second stage of labour, which is all very well for them, but it takes their eye right off what the medics are up to. You will need to keep an eye out to make sure that, where medically possible, her wishes are being respected.

* * *

Lunch has come and gone and been followed by another examination and dose of gel. This left Elle reeling, like a kick from a mule, and the exam was really painful. Not for the first time, I felt a strong desire to thump the midwife who was causing my wife such unnecessary pain – especially as this one was wearing a teddy badge and a soppy grin which suggested that her mind was far away – probably in the back of a celebrity's limo trying to prove the old story about nurses being a sure thing.

Something that isn't so sure is whether our baby's going to arrive today. After a lot of pain and prodding, Elle's back on the ward and none the wiser. The midwives keep attaching her to a machine that measures contractions and the baby's heart, then they come along at 20 minute intervals, take a look at the printout, nod their heads and say "another 20 minutes" as if she's a beef joint. I've finished my newspaper and I'm back onto the celebrity magazines. I wonder if it's too late to get down to the foyer for an autograph.

• • •

Drama, pure and simple. Firstly, the woman in the next bed, who has complained of headaches for a few days, is rushed off to have emergency brain surgery, then Elle starts having some serious contractions.

Her poor neighbour's dilemma has left Elle without a midwife – the only one on duty has disappeared with her patient in a helicopter. Why a midwife should be a useful partner during emergency brain surgery I'm not quite clear. Anyhow, the seriousness of the situation has kept us from moaning unnecessarily about Elle's increasing pain.

Sadly, a couple of hours after contractions started to kick in, complaints are no longer unnecessary. There's still no staff on the ward and Elle is suffering. I always thought there would be something quite entertaining about contractions. I pictured Elle with a look of intense concentration on her face, puffing and blowing like a miniature train, while I rubbed her back, held her hand and dealt with a volley of abuse that would make a navvy blush. But in reality they were almost as painful to watch as they were to endure, she squeezed my hand and winced and seemed to slip away from me to a higher plane of agony each time one struck, as they did with increasing regularity, recording sharply on the monitor like tremors.

We rang the emergency buzzer and someone came to tell us that the staff were changing over and wouldn't be around for about an hour. Changing over? An hour? These people aren't manning a nuclear submarine, for Christ's sake, they're attending to the incredibly similar needs of a ward of women. And yet, despite the fact that this obviously isn't rocket science, they do seem to take a scientific approach to having a coffee and a gossip. If only I had a rocket.

Meanwhile, Elle's suffering is getting worse and I've had enough. I know I'm not the only person in the world whose partner has suffered in labour, but to be frank, I don't give a shit about anyone else. It's time for someone to act.

"Do you know who I am?"

Complaining and coping in an emergency

So what happens when things really do go wrong? If your partner is in pain it isn't easy calmly waiting your turn to be seen. But it's equally hard for the midwives to have their agenda set by whichever father-to-be shouts the loudest. You have to step back and trust the judgement of the professionals. They might be overworked, they might be tired and unsympathetic, but they are the experts. If you're really uncomfortable with the treatment your partner is getting then complain, but be firm, insistent and polite. Don't shout, and don't threaten to sue, mainly because you'll feel like a total prick afterwards.

•   •   •

Relief comes in many forms, and ours has come in the shape of a small, angry-looking midwife from the North East. After finally emerging from her lengthy handover she took one look at Elle's chart and said she was ready to go down to the delivery suite. She then attempted another examination and that's when the problems started.

Elle's hip mobility has worsened so much since the first use of the induction gel that now she can barely move her legs without yelping with pain. The contractions were like a picnic compared to this experience. The midwife seemed to get frustrated with her, then remembered herself and became more sympathetic when she saw that Elle was really unhappy.

By this stage I was totally redundant, I had tears of frustration in my eyes and I could barely look at the pain on Elle's face. I had to do something, though, and mumbled that I didn't see how Elle was going to be able to squeeze this baby out of legs clamped tighter than a nun's at an orgy. The midwife agreed, more or less, and finally said out loud what we'd been thinking for a while – Elle was going to need a Caesarean.

Another slice of life

Surgery and Caesarean sections

Despite a lot of crap in the media about the 'too posh to push' generation, most women I know would much rather have a natural labour. It
isn't hard to see why – a major operation, a great big scar and no driving or lifting for six weeks as opposed to a few – albeit agonising –
hours of pushing, puffing and panting. Most men I know would rather
see their partners undergo something 'natural' instead of being
cut open.

Caesarean sections are 'bad' because they are expensive for hospitals,
but in many cases they are a vital emergency option. A true emergency
c-section would normally be done because of a major complication in
labour, and would be carried out under general anaesthetic, which is
scary in itself, and is made worse by the fact that the man is not
allowed into the operating theatre. An elective c-section, where there
is no immediate medical danger, is normally done under local anaesthetic and you can be present throughout.

Now there's another agonising wait while the powers that
be fart about trying to decide whether Elle should actually be allowed the operation that she so clearly needs. But

what she also needs is a painkiller, as the contractions are still coming hard and fast. She can't have anything until they've made a decision on the c-section.

To ease the pain, the staff have at least allowed Elle to hobble down to the delivery suite. Every movement seems to be agonising, from the closing of the lift door to the jolt as it finishes its descent. I'm done with being meek now, I'm not going to tolerate any other course of action, even though I have absolutely no idea whether this is the best thing for her.

My concern is, in part, selfish. I don't want to see any more of this pain. I know now that I would have really struggled with the idea of a natural labour. It is very embarrassing to note how easily I've crumbled into a desire to fix everything quickly. But as far as I can see, nothing means more than the here and now and I'm scared, for her, for me, for the baby.

•   •   •

Everything else is a blur. Well, that's not strictly true, it's all here in my memory, but it was so bizarre and dreamlike I can only tell it in a slightly amazed retrospect, as if explaining the plot of some fantastic film I've just seen.

The story, in a nutshell, is this: couple arrive at delivery suite, close to tears and state of collapse, yet ready for a fight. Fiery and scary Geordie midwife leans on quiet delivery suite midwife until caesarean becomes only option, midwife speaks to senior doctor on duty who agrees to operation. Forms are filled in, serious talk is given and husband is sent out to get baby's gear from boot of car. All in the space of about half an hour.

As far as I could make out, the male lead in this drama was played by this bloke who had a split personality. On the one hand, he thought that he was some sort of medical expert – he got himself dressed up in a blue suit with a weird shower cap and rinsed his hands, shaking the water droplets off in the time honoured senior surgeon style. On the other hand, the same bloke was reduced to a grinning, grimacing wreck, forced to sit in humiliated silence on a garden chair in the corner of a room while his wife was prepared for an operation.

Like all movies, the reality of this was a lot duller than the image – Elle's bed was wheeled into a room that looked like some kind of workshop, I guessed it was a side room that they used as a holding bay for pre-op women. A paint spattered beat box was playing some tinny Robbie Williams songs in the background. I half expected the caretaker to come in and start washing his brushes in the sink.

They got poor Elle sitting up and moaned that she couldn't get her legs high enough for the injection into her spine. Everyone, even the struggling anaesthetist, seemed too relaxed. I wasn't relaxed and I was wearing a blue suit, the type that surgeons wear.

Then the senior doctor who had given the go-ahead for the operation came in, dressed in gear almost as important looking as mine, and starting getting ready to operate. This was the stage where I could have stopped him, demanded to see his ID card, certificates etc. I could have got him to try a practice cut somewhere discreet, so that I could check out how steady his hand was. Was that alcohol I smelt on his breath? No, it was being spread all over Elle's back, a weird kind of cherry brandy-like substance. But not, I guessed – by now familiar with the medical world – actually cherry brandy.

The spinal block was giving them some gip, and another anaesthetist was paged, just like in real life medical TV drama shows. I began to worry that the staff had over-stretched themselves. But right at the last minute the anaesthetist managed to get the needle in, what a genius. All was ready.

A small windbreak was set up to protect Elle from the sight of her soon-to-be open belly, and I was allowed to shuffle my plastic chair over to be with her. She was shivering uncontrollably and suddenly I thought something dreadful must be wrong. I looked around at all the medical people getting on with their jobs and whimpered something about Elle's shaking. Don't worry, it's normal they all replied, automatically, each one of them thinking 'get this tosser out of the theatre'. Even though it resembled a tatty broom cupboard, a theatre it well and truly was. And just to hammer the point home, the surgeon started to cut.

I quickly developed a nasty case of tennis fan's neck, switching my attention between Elle's anxious face and the surgeon's intense concentration. Was that a twinge of pain? No, 15 love. Was that a look of concern? No, 15 all.

He called for forceps. Is that good? Yes, I think so, 15-30. He disappeared and grunted with huge effort. Was he struggling to free the baby? It didn't seem so, 15-40.

A thin, low, slightly pathetic cry and the game was over. The surgeon had won, and he was holding a trophy high in the air, a deep pink trophy with a purple umbilical cord twisting like a phone flex.

His assistant beamed down at us. "Do you want to know what it is?"

"No," I replied, "We want to wait until its 18th birthday. What do you think, you stupid bitch."

"Yes," I replied, cowering next to my shivering wife.

"It's a boy," she said.

Of course it is. How could it possibly be anything else? Only a boy can become lifelong captain of the England football and cricket teams. Only a tough, rough little male can be a virile, sexually active yet charming and responsible Romeo with a penis like a fire hose. The minute I saw him, this scrawny, crumpled rag of a boy, I knew he was going to be the first emperor of the known universe. And I knew that I'd always really known that, to tell the truth.

Back to that penis again. While they were getting Elle stitched up, the midwife took me and the boy through the rivers of blood and gunk into the recovery room, where she dressed him while I stood giggling quietly by her side.

No guts, no glory
Coping with all that blood

All the blood and other strange fluid is common in almost all types of delivery, and it can be a bit scary, but now is not the time to scream 'what have you done?' and fling yourself protectively across your partner's body. The trick is to take your lead from the attitude and expressions of the midwives, or the doctors. They have a habit of being brusque and professional, but when things go wrong they'll get worried just like anyone. So whatever's happening around you, if they are calm, stay calm.

The assistant in this room glanced across at us and asked about the baby's sex. "It's a boy," the midwife said. "A well-endowed boy."

"Takes after his father," I said, quick as a flash. What took a little longer was the slow realisation that this comment seemed to suggest I was either: A. hitting on an elderly midwife minutes after my wife had given birth; B. boasting about my penis in a juvenile and plainly untrue manner; or C. talking out of my arse.

As it turned out, my cock and bull story passed without comment from either woman, and I was able to collapse into another plastic chair, holding my son for the first time. God, he looked awful. He didn't look as bad as some of those freakish babies with heads like ice cream cones, or ones with faces like gargoyles, but he did have a lot of blood and mess on him and though my natural instinct was to kiss him tenderly, my gut reaction said he'd be much better off with a firm handshake.

It was all over pretty quickly after that. They wheeled Elle in and took our picture, marvelling at the quality of our camera. By now I was taking every compliment as personal approval of my manhood, so I just beamed with huge pride and a little embarrassment for the sake of the lesser men in the room. Just before we went back up to the ward, I was made to go and take off my dressing-up clothes. In the prep room, there was another dad-to-be getting ready. I walked up to him, laughing amiably, patted him on the shoulder and assured him everything would be just great. And to be fair, for his part, he looked at me as if I was a complete tosser.

Then it was back to the ward – a side ward without awful sick people thank God – a quick kiss goodnight for my family and, as the credits rolled, I was unceremoniously packed off home.

Driving through the dead streets at 1am, it felt like I was on a different planet. But I suppose I am – I'm on planet parenthood, a bizarre world where everyone talks like idiots and where visiting a family fun pub seems like a good idea. I only hope I'm going to like it here.

•   •   •

Back down here on Earth I've just called the new grand-parents and my closest friend. Not everyone was entirely understanding of my witless babbling, which I can't help as I'm so very, very tired. I had trouble remembering the key details of birth weight, exact time of delivery, eye colour and family resemblances. He still doesn't have a name, either. If I was alert enough to care, I'd probably feel sorry for our poor families, sitting and waiting at the other end of a phone line, not knowing the drama that's just unfolded. But I need to eat, drink a large glass of something alcoholic and go to bed with a good book. I should be worried that I'll have trouble sleeping, that I'll just replay the day's events over and over in my head. But to be honest, I wouldn't believe it had happened.

•   •   •

After the thrills and spills of the boy's first day in the world, his second must have seemed like an anticlimax. But for me it was a much better pace. We've had the whole day together as a family, left in total isolation on the side ward. The midwives have popped in for the odd chat and to demonstrate things like bathing and feeding, but otherwise it has just been the three of us.

Elle's been a bit tired and pretty overwhelmed all day, but she's got the calm manner of someone who knows they've done a good job. She's also got the relief of rediscovering her health – as soon as the numbing effect of the anaesthetic wore off, she realised that her mobility problems had seriously faded. For the first time in weeks, she walked without her crutches. It might not seem like much, but it feels like a minor miracle.

The decision to keep our families at bay was one of the toughest, but best choices we've made. Of course, it depends on them respecting our privacy – they could have just turned up today unannounced, but they've left us to it, though Elle's parents must be itching to see their first grandchild. The effect has been that I've taken my first few steps into fatherhood without fear of judgement or criticism. The family will get their chance to meet the new arrival next week, when we're back in a familiar place with an established routine.

Getting home is so important to Elle, who is now really sick of the hospital. To start off with we'd thought that she might spend a couple of days in a smaller, community hospital run by midwives, but the whole experience has put her right off healthcare. She's begged the powers that be to let her out as soon as possible, and I've promised I'll be on hand to look after her and the boy. They've agreed to an early parole.

Tomorrow I get to drive my wife and son home for the first time. I've spent hours testing the fittings on the child seat, and I'm just about happy with it. I'm nervous and full of pride and anticipation.

So far he's spent most of his time asleep, which is understandable given his sudden and dramatic entry to the world. But he's shown us enough of his little personality to road-test his new name, and it seems to stick.

So it's a big welcome to Oliver. Good luck mate. With a dad like me, you're going to need it.

Epilogue
Merry Xmas everybody

If someone had told me last Christmas that I'd be celebrating this year with my new son, I'd have laughed them all the way to the lunatic asylum. Yet a few short weeks after the traumatic, stunning and amazing events of my son's birth it is Christmas again, and life has come around in a full circle as dizzying as any carousel. And despite all the strangeness, somehow it feels as if this is how life has always been.

There have always been stinking nappies and fountains of pee, tiny clothes dripping on the line, huge supermarket bills, endless visits from cooing, soppy grandparents, sleepless nights and exhausted days. There have always been old-aged midwives and new age health visitors, doctors' appointments, frightening baby jabs and endless weighing sessions. There's always been a house crammed to the roof with plastic toys and fluffy bears. There's always been the dilemma between being a good father and becoming a control freak.

But that's all a different story. This one has come to its happy end.

Contact us

You're welcome to contact White Ladder Press if you have any questions or comments for either us or the authors. Please use whichever of the following routes suits you.

Phone: **0208 334 1600**

Email: **enquiries@whiteladderpress.com**

Fax: **0208 334 1601**

Address: **2nd Floor, Westminster House, Kew Road, Richmond, Surrey TW9 2ND**

Website: **www.whiteladderpress.com**

What can our website do for you?

If you want more information about any of our books, you'll find it at **www.whiteladderpress.com**. In particular you'll find extracts from each of our books, and reviews of those that are already published. We also run special offers on future titles if you order online before publication. And you can request a copy of our free catalogue.

Many of our books have links pages, useful addresses and so on relevant to the subject of the book. You'll also find out a bit more about us and, if you're a writer yourself, you'll find our submission guidelines for authors. So please check us out and let us know if you have any comments, questions or suggestions.

You're the Daddy

The ultimate guide to being a new Dad for blokes

Stephen Giles

"The perfect gift for a soon-to-be or new dad. It's a great read."
Parenting Magazine

New dad? Or about to be? Good for you. The best thing in the world, and all that. Now life can get back to normal, right? Well, kind of…

You're The Daddy explains what life will really be like from here on. Written by Stephen Giles (who also wrote From Lad to Dad, The ultimate guide to pregnancy for blokes), it's crammed with information and practical tips. It's easy to read, funnier than most of your mates, and explains all the important stuff you'll need to know to get you through the next year, such as:

- **Sleep** You're probably realising why sleep deprivation is used as a torture. What can you expect your baby to do, when, and how can you cope?
- **Sex** when does this start again, and does breastfeeding really work as a contraceptive? And when and how can you get your relationship with your partner back?
- **Cash** You know you spent a small fortune before the baby was born? Well, there's more – but how much more? And are there solutions which don't involve sending your baby out to sweep chimneys?
- **Your Baby** Right now the fruit of even your loins probably doesn't do much more than sleep and poo. Just what can you expect them to do and when?

Stephen will help you ensure that by the end of your first year not only will you be able to change a nappy in your sleep (should you be lucky enough to get any) but, more importantly, you'll have mastered the art of being a great dad.

£8.99